OXFOR

# Pulmonary Arterial Hypertension

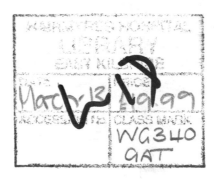

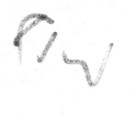

# O C L
OXFORD CARDIOLOGY LIBRARY

# Pulmonary Arterial Hypertension

Edited by

## Professor Michael A Gatzoulis

Royal Brompton Hospital and National Heart
and Lung Institute, Imperial College, London, UK

## OXFORD
UNIVERSITY PRESS

# OXFORD
UNIVERSITY PRESS

Great Clarendon Street, Oxford, OX2 6DP,
United Kingdom

Oxford University Press is a department of the University of Oxford.
It furthers the University's objective of excellence in research, scholarship,
and education by publishing worldwide. Oxford is a registered trade mark of
Oxford University Press in the UK and in certain other countries

British Library Cataloguing in Publication Data
Data available

Library of Congress Cataloging in Publication Data
Data available

ISBN 978-0-19-957263-2

Printed in Great Britain by
Clays Ltd, St Ives plc

# Contents

# Preface

Pulmonary arterial hypertension (PAH) is no longer an orphan disease. Only a decade or two ago PAH used to carry a grave prognosis, the diagnosis was often very delayed, and it was mostly young patients presenting at advanced stages who were inflicted. Recent improvements in our understanding of the disease and, in particular, recent advances in therapy mean that now, these patients have gone from a state of no hope to one where prolonged survival coupled with improved quality of life are the norm. *It is, therefore, timely to visit this increasingly important area and provide a concise background and a state of the art approach towards the diagnosis and management of PAH for medical and allied professionals, who may not be fully emerged in the field.*

I am indebted to our wonderful faculty, leading PAH experts from the UK and around the world, for donating their precious time to produce excellent chapters and make this small textbook a reality. I am also grateful to Eloise Moir-Ford and the Oxford University Press Team for their help, patience and support, which was essential for carrying the project through in a timely fashion.

While it is hoped that this book will improve early diagnosis and appropriate management for patients with PAH, it remains a challenge for us all to improve further our understanding of the precise PAH aetiology and, thus, be able to develop specific aetiologic therapies to combat this devastating disease.

Professor Michael A Gatzoulis

*To my parents and my teachers at the 8th Primary & The Boys Grammar School in Drama and at the Aristotelian Medical School in Thessaloniki, Greece.*

# Foreword

Our improved understanding of pulmonary arterial hypertension (PAH) and recent advances in therapy present us with the obvious challenge of spreading this ever-increasing knowledge to a broader professional audience, which in turn will we hope improve prognosis for our patients.

I am delighted to write the forward for this concise pocket volume, providing both essential and easily accessible information for the non-tertiary PAH health care professional in the *Oxford Cardiology Library* tradition of the series. Professor Gatzoulis from the Royal Brompton Hospital, the editor of the book, has compiled a comprehensive text, inviting expertise from UK and world authorities in the PAH field. The book outlines the key points with respect to the latest classification, pathobiology, genetics, clinical assessment of the patient with suspected PAH and the role of imaging. There are specific chapters addressing different PAH aetiologies, namely idiopathic PAH, thromboembolic PAH, PAH related to connective tissue disease, congenital heart disease (Eisenmenger complex), respiratory disease and other unusual causes. Last, but not least, the book addresses counselling, contraception and the latest therapy for the challenging area of pregnancy and PAH, which is still associated with a high maternal mortality risk.

The main objective of the book is to increase awareness of PAH, promote rapid diagnostic work up and timely specialist referral so that effective therapy is made available as early as possible to all patients with suspected or known PAH. I believe that every physician, nurse or other health care professional—whether senior or junior—who may encounter patients with PAH has much to gain from this book.

Professor Dame Carol Black

# List of contributors

**Elisabeth Bédard, MD FRCPC**
Consultant Cardiologist,
University Institute of
Cardiology and Pneumology of
Quebec,
Quebec City, Quebec, Canada.

**Craig S Broberg, MD FACC**
Director,
Adult Congenital Heart
Program,
Oregon Health and Science
University,
Portland, OR, USA.

**Chien-Nien Chen**
PhD Student,
Clinical Pharmacology and
Investigative Sciences,
Imperial College, London, UK.

**Natali AY Chung, MD MRCP**
Consultant Cardiologist,
Adult Congenital Heart Disease,
Guy's and St Thomas' NHS
Foundation Trust,
London, UK.

**J Gerry Coghlan, MD**
Consultant Cardiologist and
Clinical Lead,
Pulmonary Hypertension,
Royal Free Hospital,
London, UK.

**Tamera Jo Corte, MBBS Bsc(Med), FRACP, PhD**
Consultant Respiratory Physician,
Royal Prince Alfred Hospital,
and University of Sydney,
Sydney, Australia.

**Stephen F Crawley, MBChB**
Clinical Research Fellow,
Scottish Pulmonary Vascular
Unit,
Glasgow, UK.

**Konstantinos Dimopoulos, MD, PhD, FESC**
Consultant Cardiologist,
Adult Congenital Heart Centre
and Centre for Pulmonary
Hypertension,
Royal Brompton Hospital,
and the National Heart & Lung
Institute,
Imperial College,
London, UK.

**Michael A Gatzoulis, MD, PhD, FACC, FESC**
Professor of Cardiology,
Congenital Heart Disease and
Consultant Cardiologist,
Adult Congenital Heart Centre
and Centre for Pulmonary
Hypertension,
Royal Brompton Hospital, and
the National Heart & Lung
Institute,
Imperial College,
London, UK.

**Georgios Giannakoulas, MD**
Consultant Cardiologist,
1st Department of Cardiology,
AHEPA Hospital,
Aristotle University of
Thessaloniki,
Greece.

**Sara Goletto, MD**
Consultant Cardiologist,
Azienda Ospedaliera della
Provincia di Lodi,
Italy.

**Mark D Hiatt, MD, MBA, MS**
Consultant Radiologist,
Trinity Mother Frances
Hospitals & Clinics,
Tyler, TX, USA.

**Ryo Inuzuka, MD**
Department of Adult
Congenital Heart Disease and
Pediatrics,
Chiba Cardiovascular Center,
Chiba, Japan.

**David P Jenkins, FRCS**
Lead Surgeon,
National Pulmonary
Endarterectomy Programme,
Consultant Cardiac and
Transplant Surgeon,
Papworth Hospital NHS
Foundation Trust,
Cambridge, UK.

**Michael J Landzberg, MD**
Founder and Director,
Boston Adult Congenital
Heart (BACH) and Pulmonary
Hypertension Service,
Children's Hospital Boston,
Brigham and Women's
Hospital,
Harvard Medical School,
Boston, MA, USA.

**Rajiv D Machado**
Senior Fellow,
Molecular and Medical Genetics
Group,
Division of Genetics &
Molecular Medicine,
Kings College,
London, UK.

**Nicholas W Morrell, MD FRCP**
British Heart Foundation
Professor of Cardiopulmonary
Medicine,
Department of Medicine,
University of Cambridge School
of Clinical Medicine,
Addenbrooke's and Papworth
Hospitals
Cambridge, UK.

**Koichiro Niwa, MD, FACC**
Director,
Department of Adult Congenital
Heart Disease and Pediatrics,
Chiba Cardiovascular Center,
Chiba, Japan.

**Alexander R Opotowsky, MD, MPH**
Boston Adult Congenital Heart
and Pulmonary Hypertension
Service,
Children's Hospital Boston,
Brigham and Women's Hospital,
Harvard Medical School,
Boston, MA, USA.

**Andrew J Peacock, MD, FRCP**
Professor and Consultant
Respiratory Physician,
Director,
Scottish Pulmonary Vascular
Unit,
Golden Jubilee National
Hospital,
Glasgow, UK.

**Joanna Pepke-Zaba, PhD, FRCP**
Director,
National Pulmonary Vascular Diseases Unit,
Consultant in Respiratory Medicine,
Papworth Hospital NHS Foundation Trust,
Cambridge, UK.

**Benji E Schreiber, MBBS, MRCP**
Consultant in Rheumatology & General Medicine,
Pulmonary Hypertension,
Department of Cardiology,
Royal Free Hospital,
London, UK.

**Karen Sheares, FRCP**
Consultant Respiratory Physician,
Pulmonary Hypertension,
Papworth Hospital NHS Foundation Trust,
Cambridge, UK.

**Richard C Trembath, FMedSci**
Professor and Head of Molecular and
Medical Genetics Group,
Division of Genetics & Molecular Medicine,
Kings College,
London, UK.

**Christopher J Valerio, MBBS, MRCP**
Pulmonary Hypertension,
Department of Cardiology,
Royal Free Hospital,
London, UK.

**Martin R Wilkins, MD**
Professor of Clinical Pharmacology,
Head of the Division of Investigative Sciences,
Imperial College
and Director of the Clinical and Investigative Sciences within Imperial College Healthcare NHS Trust,
London, UK.

**S John Wort, MD, FRCP**
Consultant and Clinical Lead in Pulmonary Hypertension,
Royal Brompton Hospital, and the National Heart & Lung Institute,
Imperial College,
London, UK.

**Zhenguo Zhai, MD**
Visiting Fellow,
Clinical Pharmacology and Investigative Sciences,
Imperial College,
London, UK.

**Lan Zhao, MD**
Lecturer in Clinical Pharmacology and Investigative Sciences,
Imperial College,
London, UK.

# Abbreviations

| | |
|---|---|
| ACHD | adult population of patients with congenital heart disease |
| AM | adrenomedullin |
| ANA | anti-nuclear antibodies |
| ANP | atrial natriuretic peptide |
| APAH | associated pulmonary arterial hypertension |
| aPL | antiphospholipid antibodies |
| ART | antiretroviral therapy |
| ASD | atrial septal defects |
| AVM | arterio-venous malformations |
| BLT | bilateral lung transplantation |
| BMP | bone morphorgenetic protein |
| BNP | B-type natriuretic peptide |
| BSA | body surface area |
| CCB | calcium channel blockers |
| CF | cystic fibrosis |
| CI | cardiac index |
| CPB | cardiopulmonary bypass |
| CO | cardiac output |
| COPD | chronic obstructive pulmonary disease |
| CPET | cardiopulmonary exercise tests |
| CREST | calcinosis, Raynaud's phenomenon, oesophageal dysmotility, sclerodactyly, and telangiectasia |
| CT | computed tomography |
| CTD | connective tissue diseases |
| CTDPAH | connective tissue disease associated pulmonary arterial hypertension |
| CTEPH | chronic thromboembolic pulmonary hypertension |
| CVP | central venous pressure |
| CXR | chest x-ray |
| DCA | dichloroacetate |
| DCSSc | diffuse cutaneous systemic sclerosis |
| DHCA | deep hypothermic circulatory arrest |

| DLco | low diffusing capacity for carbon monoxide |
| dPAP | diastolic pulmonary artery pressure |
| dsDNA | double-stranded DNA |
| DVT | deep vein thrombosis |
| ECG | electrocardiogram |
| ECMO | extracorporeal membrane oxygenation |
| eNOS | endothelial nitric oxide synthase |
| ERA | endothelin receptor antagonist |
| ETA | endothelin type A |
| ETB | endothelin type B |
| GAVE | gastric antral vascular ectasia |
| HCX | pulmonary histiocytosis X |
| HHT | hereditary haemorrhagic telangiectasia |
| HIV | human immunodeficiency virus |
| HPAH | heritable pulmonary arterial hypertension |
| HPV | hypoxic pulmonary vasoconstriction |
| HR | heart rate |
| ILD | interstitial lung disease |
| IPAH | idiopathic pulmonary arterial hypertension |
| IPF | idiopathic pulmonary fibrosis |
| IVC | inferior vena cava |
| LA | left atrium |
| LAM | lymphangioleiomyomatosis |
| LCH | Langerhans cell histiocytosis |
| LCSSc | limited cutaneous systemic sclerosis |
| LV | left ventricle |
| MAP | mean systemic arterial pressure |
| MCTD | mixed connective tissue disease |
| mPAP | mean pulmonary arterial pressure |
| MRI | magnetic resonance imaging |
| NFAT | nuclear factor of activated T cells |
| NMD | nonsense-mediated decay |
| NO | nitric oxide |
| NYHA | New York Heart Association |
| OHS | obesity hypoventilation syndrome |
| oPAH | PAH due to other causes |
| OPG | osteoprotegerin |

| | |
|---|---|
| OSA | obstructive sleep apnoea |
| PA | pulmonary arterial |
| PAH | pulmonary arterial hypertension |
| PAOP | pulmonary artery occlusion pressure |
| PAP | pulmonary artery pressure |
| PASP | pulmonary artery systolic pressure |
| PCWP | pulmonary capillary wedge pressure |
| PDA | patent ductus arteriosus |
| PDGF | platelet-derived growth factor |
| PDGFR | platelet derived growth factor receptor |
| PE | pulmonary embolism |
| PEA | pulmonary endarterectomy |
| PFO | patent foramen ovale |
| PFT | pulmonary function tests |
| PH | pulmonary hypertension |
| PVR | pulmonary vascular resistance |
| PVRi | pulmonary vascular resistance indexed to BSA |
| RA | rheumatoid arthritis |
| RA | right atrium |
| RANK | receptor activator of nuclear factor-B |
| RANKL | RANK ligand |
| RHC | right heart catheter |
| RV | right ventricle |
| RVOT | RV outflow tract |
| 6MWT | 6 minute walk test |
| SLE | systemic lupus erythematosus |
| SLT | single lung transplantation |
| sPAP | systolic pulmonary artery pressure |
| SS | Sjögren's syndrome |
| SSc | systemic sclerosis |
| SV | stroke volume |
| SVC | superior vena cava |
| SVi | stroke volume index |
| SVR | systemic vascular resistance |
| TAPSE | tricuspid annular plane systolic excursion |
| TR | tricuspid regurgitation |
| TRAIL | tumour necrosis factor-related apoptosis-inducing ligand |

| | |
|---|---|
| TV | tricuspid valve |
| UTR | untranslated region |
| VEGF | vascular endothelial growth factor |
| VIP | vasoactive intestinal peptide |
| VSD | ventricular septal defects |
| VTE | venous thromboembolism |
| WHO | World Health Organization |
| WU | Wood unit |

## Chapter 1

# Classification of pulmonary arterial hypertension and current therapeutic approach

Natali AY Chung and Michael A Gatzoulis

**Key points**

- Early diagnosis
- Classification affects therapeutic approach
- Importance of multidisciplinary approach and supportive therapy
- Advanced treatment options.

## 1.1 Definition and diagnosis of pulmonary arterial hypertension

Pulmonary arterial hypertension (PAH) involves pulmonary vascular remodelling with luminal obliteration of small vessels, resultant raised pulmonary vascular resistance and ultimately right ventricular failure and death. There are numerous conditions associated with raised pulmonary arterial pressure but overall morbidity and mortality remains high (Figure 1.1).

### 1.1.1 Definition of pulmonary arterial hypertension

Normal mean pulmonary artery pressure is 11–17 mmHg, although there is some variation with age and weight. PAH is defined as a sustained mean pulmonary arterial pressure (mPAP) of >25 mmHg at rest in the presence of normal left-sided cardiac pressures reflected by a pulmonary capillary wedge pressure or left ventricular end diastolic pressure of ≤15 mmHg. Moreover, pulmonary vascular resistance should be ≥3 mmHg/l/min (Woods units) or 240 dynes/s/cm5.

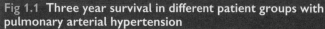

Fig 1.1 **Three year survival in different patient groups with pulmonary arterial hypertension**

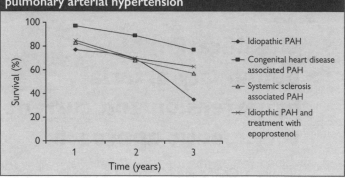

Legend:
- Idiopathic PAH
- Congenital heart disease associated PAH
- Systemic sclerosis associated PAH
- Idiopthic PAH and treatment with epoprostenol

X-axis: Time (years)
Y-axis: Survival (%)

## 1.1.2 Symptomatic presentation

The clinical presentation of PAH can be very variable and often non-specific. Main symptoms include breathlessness, chest pain, palpitations, and syncope. The severity of symptoms can be described according to the World Health Organization (WHO) Functional Classification 1998 (Figure 1.2). This is a particularly useful tool both in the initial assessment of patients and in the monitoring of disease progression over time or in response to therapy. Studies have shown that survival of idiopathic PAH is poor, with a median survival of 2.8 years after diagnosis, emphasizing the importance of prompt diagnosis.

Fig 1.2 **Functional classification of pulmonary hypertension according to World Health Organization 1998**

**Class I:** Patients with pulmonary hypertension but without resulting limitation of physical activity. Ordinary physical activity does not cause undue dyspnoea or fatigue, chest pain, or near syncope.

**Class II:** Patients with pulmonary hypertension resulting in slight limitation of physical activity. They are comfortable at rest. Ordinary physical activity causes undue dyspnoea or fatigue, chest pain, or near syncope.

**Class III:** Patients with pulmonary hypertension resulting in marked limitation of physical activity. They are comfortable at rest. Less than ordinary physical activity causes undue dyspnoea or fatigue, chest pain, or near syncope.

**Class IV:** Patients with pulmonary hypertension with inability to carry out physical activity without symptoms. These patients manifest signs of right heart failure. Dyspnoea and/or fatigue may even be present at rest. Discomfort is increased by any physical activity.

## 1.2 **Classification of pulmonary arterial hypertension**

PAH may be an isolated finding or associated with numerous conditions. As discussed in the next chapter many of the underlying pathological findings in PAH are consistent with vascular proliferation and remodelling, regardless of aetiology.

PAH was previously divided simplistically into primary or secondary, the diagnosis of primary PAH being one of exclusion. However, there are a great many causes or associations with PAH resulting in the five categories of the Evian classification in 1998 which was based on specific therapeutic approaches. The most recent modification of this classification (in Dana Point, 2008) was based on new understandings of disease mechanisms (Table 1.1). This is a clinical classification which groups together causative diseases according to similar clinical presentations, pathophysiology and treatment options. This revised classification provides the current framework for understanding PAH.

## 1.3 **Therapeutic approaches**

### 1.3.1 **Early diagnosis**

Due to the non-specific presentation of PAH patients are often diagnosed at a considerable period after their initial presentation, often over one year. More non-specific clinical presentations may include atypical chest pain, fatigue and dizziness. Clinical suspicion should be high in those with predisposing conditions for PAH (see Table 1.1) and where appropriate patients should have regular screening for raised pulmonary artery systolic pressure by transthoracic echocardiography. However, one should also be suspicious in those with breathlessness with no overt cardiac or pulmonary disease.

The clinical signs include a right ventricular heave, loud pulmonary component to the second heart sound, and murmurs of tricuspid regurgitation or pulmonary regurgitation. More advanced findings include cool peripheries, raised jugular venous pulse, hepatomegaly, and abdominal ascites in keeping with right heart failure. Easily accessible, non-invasive investigations of ECG and CXR are abnormal in the majority of patients.

### 1.3.2 **Multidisciplinary approach**

The assessment, diagnosis, and treatment of pulmonary hypertension can be a daunting and complex route for patients. Moreover, the impact of symptoms on day-to-day living and the reality of

## Table 1.1 Updated clinical classification of pulmonary hypertension (Dana Point, 2008[1])

**1 Pulmonary arterial hypertension (PAH)**
- 1.1 Idiopathic
- 1.2 Heritable
    - 1.2.1 BMPR2
    - 1.2.2 ALK1, endoglin (with or without hereditary haemorrhagic telangiectasia)
    - 1.2.3 Unknown
- 1.3 Drugs and toxins induced
- 1.4 Associated with (APAH)
    - 1.4.1 Connective tissue diseases
    - 1.4.2 HIV infection
    - 1.4.3 Portal hypertension
    - 1.4.4 Congenital heart disease
    - 1.4.5 Schistosomiasis
    - 1.4.6 Chronic haemolytic anaemia
- 1.5 Persistent pulmonary hypertension of the newborn

**1′ Pulmonary veno-occlusive disease and/or pulmonary capillary haemangiomatosis**

**2 Pulmonary hypertension due to left heart disease**
- 2.1 Systolic dysfunction
- 2.2 Diastolic dysfunction
- 2.3 Valvular disease

**3 Pulmonary hypertension due to lung diseases and/or hypoxia**
- 3.1 Chronic obstructive pulmonary disease
- 3.2 Interstitial lung disease
- 3.3 Other pulmonary diseases with mixed restrictive and obstructive pattern
- 3.4 Sleep-disordered breathing
- 3.5 Alveolar hypoventilation disorders
- 3.6 Chronic exposure to high altitude
- 3.7 Developmental abnormalities

**4 Chronic thromboembolic pulmonary hypertension**

**5 PH with unclear and/or multifactorial mechanisms**
- 5.1 Haematological disorders: myeloproliferative disorders, splenectomy
- 5.2 Systemic disorders: sarcoidosis, pulmonary Langerhans cell histiocytosis, lymphangioleiomyomatosis, neurofibromatosis, vasculitis
- 5.3 Metabolic disorders: glycogen storage disease, Gaucher disease, thyroid disorders
- 5.4 Others: tumoural obstruction, fibrosing mediastinitis, chronic renal failure on dialysis

ALK-1 = activin receptor-like kinase 1 gene; APAH = associated pulmonary arterial hypertension; BMPR2 = bone morphogenetic protein receptor, type 2; HIV = human immunodeficiency virus; PAH = pulmonary arterial hypertension.

[1] Simmoneau G, Robbins IM, Beghetti M, et al. (2009). Updated clinical classification of pulmonary hypertension. *J Am Coll Cardiol* **54**: 43–54.

disease progression and prognosis can be overwhelming. Access to a multidisciplinary team can make a significant impact on the patient's journey. The collaboration between cardiologists, respiratory physicians and radiologists will expedite the timely investigation and diagnosis of patients. Moreover, once a diagnosis is made patients will need continued re-assessment to monitor the progression of disease and response to therapy.

The addition of specialist nurses to the team cannot only help facilitate the organization of this follow up, but they also provide indispensable support to patients and their families. Often patients feel isolated and uncertain about a disease which cannot be cured and which is life-shortening. Access to team members that they can discuss these issues with and who can provide contacts to patient support groups and psychological support where needed is essential (Pulmonary Hypertension Association-UK, www.phassociation.uk.com).

In the later stages of disease the early involvement of a palliative care team should be considered. The palliative care team can help provide additional approaches to symptom relief as well as dealing with end of life issues.

### 1.3.3 General measures

Patient education, advice, and lifestyle modifications are important. This includes factors such as air travel, altitude and dehydration. Routine influenza and pneumococcal vaccinations are recommended. Patients should avoid strenuous physical exercise and weight lifting, but should be encouraged to remain as active as their symptoms allow. Exercise should stop if patients develop moderate to severe breathlessness, exertional dizziness, or chest pain.

Effective contraception should be discussed with all women of childbearing age. Although maternal mortality has fallen in the last decade the overall risk is still approximately 25% and pregnancy should, therefore, only be undertaken after detailed discussion and in close collaboration with a high risk cardiac obstetric service. Oestrogens should be avoided due to the increased risk of thrombosis.

### 1.3.4 Supportive medical therapy

#### 1.3.4.1 Anticoagulation

As well as thromboembolic disease being a cause of pulmonary hypertension, in situ thrombosis is a recognized pathological finding in PAH. This is thought to be associated with demonstrated abnormalities of the coagulation and fibrinolytic pathways as well as platelet dysfunction. To date anticoagulation has only been shown to reduce mortality in those patients with idiopathic PAH (IPAH) and is recommended in this patient group. The use of warfarin in other groups should be considered, particularly if there is documented evidence of thromboembolic disease. Other indications for anticoagulation might include sustained arrhythmias or significant ventricular impairment. Uncertainty still exists in PAH in association with congenital heart disease, a group that can have both thrombotic and bleeding abnormalities.

It should be remembered that many of these patients will have a secondary erythrocytosis and raised haematocrit requiring the use of citrate adjusted sampling tubes at the time of phlebotomy to achieve an accurate coagulation profile. Liaison with the local haematology service is recommended.

### 1.3.4.2 Oxygen

There are no long-term studies to demonstrate a beneficial effect from oxygen. However, it is known to acutely reduce pulmonary vascular resistance and patients receive symptomatic benefit. Ambulatory oxygen may be prescribed in the presence of symptomatic benefit and in the presence of reversible exercise-induced desaturation. Oxygen may also be prescribed in keeping with British Thoracic Society guidelines for long term oxygen use (at least 15 hours a day) when $PaO_2$ is consistently <8kPa during a period of clinical stability or nocturnally if mean nocturnal oxygen saturations are <90%. It should be noted that patients with Eisenmenger's syndrome or chronic cyanosis clearly represent a distinct group. Every effort should be made to ensure the empirical use of oxygen does not compromise patients' daily physical activity and further contribute towards physical deconditioning.

### 1.3.4.3 Iron supplementation

Despite raised haemoglobin levels in chronic cyanosis, patients with PAH are often iron depleted. Secondary erythrocytosis in response to hypoxia results in the increased utilization of iron stores. Iron studies should, therefore, be checked in all patients and oral iron supplementation started as required. Intravenous iron can be administered if oral therapy fails. This simple therapeutic manoeuvre can dramatically improve symptom severity.

The use of venesection in response to a raised haematocrit is no longer advocated as it contributes to iron deficiency, impairs oxygen transport capacity and increases the risk of stroke. It should only be considered in the presence of true hyperviscosity symptoms.

### 1.3.4.4 Diuretics and anti-arrhythmics

Nearly all patients will require the use of regular diuretics to control symptoms associated with mainly right sided heart failure, although there are no randomized controlled trials supporting its use.

The routine use of digoxin is no longer advocated as there have been no long-term trials to support chronic therapy. It may be used as an anti-arrhythmic if suitable. Tachyarrhythmias are generally poorly tolerated and prompt identification of the arrhythmia and commencement of appropriate treatment is important.

### *1.3.4.5 Calcium channel blockers*

High dose calcium channel blockers (CCB) have been shown to be of benefit in a small group of patients with PAH. Treatment should only be initiated in those who demonstrate a positive reversibility study on right heart catheterization and who have idiopathic PAH, familial PAH or anorexigen associated PAH. The definition of a positive response is defined as a fall in mPAP ≥10 mmHg, to a mPAP ≤40 mmHg, with an unchanged or increased cardiac output. Of note, long-term responders to high dose CCB represent <10% of patients assessed in a pulmonary vascular referral unit, with only 54% of initial responders having a sustained response. Long-acting, high dose diltiazem, nifedipine, or amlodipine is usually used.

### 1.3.5 **Disease targeted therapies**

Of the above treatments, only warfarin has been demonstrated to improve survival in patients with IPAH. However, over the past decade or so treatments targeted at specific pathophysiological pathways in PAH have been shown to be effective in improving symptoms and improving prognosis in some groups. The use of targeted therapies has mostly been studied in patients in functional class III and IV, but there are on going studies looking at earlier initiation of therapy in class II patients. Haemodynamic measurements, distance covered in 6 minute walk tests (6MWT), and WHO functional class and quality of life measures have been the main studied outcomes.

### *1.3.5.1 Prostanoids*

Prostanoids were the first group of drugs which demonstrably improved prognosis, albeit in non-randomized trials, in PAH (Figure 1.1). Randomized control trials have demonstrated improved haemodynamics, 6MWT distance and quality of life over 8 to 12-week periods of therapy.

Prostanoids are analogues of prostacyclin (prostaglandin, PGI2) which is normally released by healthy endothelial cells resulting in smooth muscle relaxation and vasodilation, as well as inhibiting platelet activation. The group includes epoprostenol, iloprost, and treprostinil (not licensed in the UK). The main disadvantage of prostanoids is their route of administration: they are mostly given intravenously, subcutaneously, or via nebulizers. Thus patients are at risk of complications from indwelling intravenous lines or painful subcutaneous injection sites. Moreover, due to the short half life of the infused drugs, infusions must be continuous with dangerous consequences from unexpected interruption of delivery. Patients must be able to manage their own infusions at home or frequent nebulizers. Common side effects associated with prostanoids are headache, abdominal pain, nausea, and vomiting, flushing and limb pain. The dose of the drug is slowly increased as tolerated.

### 1.3.5.2 Endothelin antagonists

Endothelin-1 is also produced by endothelium. It is a potent vaso-constrictor, binding to endothelin type A and B receptors (ETA and ETB) on smooth muscle cells. ETA is a pure vasoconstrictor, whereas ETB has an initial vasodilator effect via nitric oxide. Bosentan is a dual receptor antagonist and the first drug to be studied. Ambrisentan and sitaxentan are selective ETA antagonists. Sitaxentan has now been withdrawn from the market because of a potential link with an increased risk of idiosyncratic response with life-threatening liver toxicity. Due to potential hepatic effects patients require monthly liver function tests, although ambrisentan is reported to have less hepatic toxicity. Other common side effects are headache and peripheral oedema. Studies have demonstrated an improvement in haemodynamics, 6MWT, Borg dyspnoea score, quality of life measurements, and also time to clinical deterioration in patients.

### 1.3.5.3 Phosphodiesterase 5 inhibitors

By inhibiting the degradation of cyclic guanosine monophosphate (cGMP) phosphodiesterase 5 inhibitors promote vasodilation in the pulmonary vasculature. To date sildenafil is the main agent used in PAH. In a randomized, double-blind, placebo-controlled study sildenafil improved NYHA functional class, 6MWT and pulmonary artery pressures over a 12-week period.

One study compared the use of sildenafil to bosentan in a randomized double blind manner. Both treatments produced similar effect when analysed on an intention to treat basis in a mixed patient population of IPAH, connective tissue disease associated PAH and congenital shunt associated PAH.

Tadalafil is another phosphodiesterase 5 inhibitor in use; there has been a small observational study in Eisenmenger patients to demonstrate safety and efficacy and one randomized controlled trial in idopathic and associated PAH patients.

### 1.3.6 **Invasive procedures**

### 1.3.6.1 Transplantation

Single lung, double lung and lung/heart transplantation has been performed for PAH over the last 25 years. Although results from single and double lung transplants have been similar the effect of complications in single transplants has advocated a move towards double lung transplantation only. Heart lung transplantation should be considered if there is considerable involvement of the right heart which is not thought to be reversible or in the presence of congenital heart disease. It is worth remembering that the prognosis in patients with associated congenital heart disease is better than other groups and the natural history of the condition may produce better long-term results.

Transplantation should only be considered after the use of disease-targeted therapies and in those patients who remain in WHO functional class III or IV.

### 1.3.6.2 Atrial septostomy

The creation of an interatrial right to left shunt can result in off-loading of the right ventricle, increases in left ventricular preload and increases in cardiac output. It is reserved for those patients in WHO class IV, those refractory to right heart failure treatment or those with syncopal symptoms. The long-term effect of atrial septostomy is uncertain and it is used as a bridge for patients failing on medical therapy or as a palliative step. Care should be taken with patient selection as risks are greatly increased if resting oxygen saturations in air are <80% or if mean right atrial pressure is >20 mmHg.

### 1.3.6.3 Pulmonary thromboendarterectomy

This should be considered in patients with chronic thromboembolic pulmonary hypertension (CTEPH). If mPAP is >50 mmHg at the time of presentation <20% of patients survive two years. It should be noted that the procedure itself continues to be high risk with operative mortality reported at 5–15%. Patients should be referred to an appropriate centre for early assessment of operative suitability.

### 1.3.7 **Choice of therapy and combination treatment**

Patients with PAH should be referred to a designated, specialized pulmonary hypertension unit for the confirmation of diagnosis and initiation of treatment. After the institution of general measures, the choice of first line therapy remains individualized and challenging due to the wide variation in clinical practices and the range of different

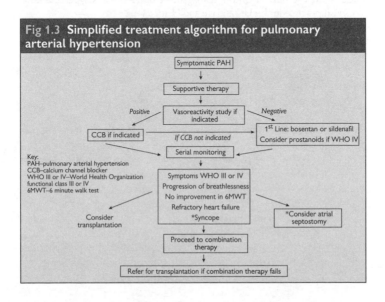

**Fig 1.3 Simplified treatment algorithm for pulmonary arterial hypertension**

Symptomatic PAH

Supportive therapy

Vasoreactivity study if indicated

Positive → CCB if indicated

Negative → 1st Line: bosentan or sildenafil Consider prostanoids if WHO IV

If CCB not indicated

Serial monitoring

Symptoms WHO III or IV
Progression of breathlessness
No improvement in 6MWT
Refractory heart failure
*Syncope

Consider transplantation

*Consider atrial septostomy

Proceed to combination therapy

Refer for transplantation if combination therapy fails

Key:
PAH–pulmonary arterial hypertension
CCB–calcium channel blocker
WHO III or IV–World Health Organization functional class III or IV
6MWT–6 minute walk test

aetiologies of PAH. Often bosentan (as the oldest endothelin antagonist) or sildenafil are used first line due to the problems associated with the administration of prostanoids. If single therapy is unsuccessful than a combination of treatments can be used, the rationale being that more than one disease pathway is targeted, in a similar approach to the treatment of systemic hypertension (Figure 1.3). Studies in this area are, however, limited and where possible patients in whom combination therapy is being considered should be enrolled into ongoing studies. In appropriate cases invasive procedures will also be considered.

# References

ACCF/AHA (2009) Expert Consensus Document on Pulmonary Hypertension. *JACC* **53**: 1573–1619.

Bédard E, Dimopoulos K, Gatzoulis MA (2009) Has there been any progress made on pregnancy outcomes among women with pulmonary arterial hypertension? *Eur Heart J* **30**(3): 256–65.

Diller G, Gatzoulis MA (2007) Pulmonary vascular disease in adults with congenital heart disease. *Circ* **115**: 1039–50.

Galie *et al.* on behalf of the Task Force for Diagnosis and Treatment of Pulmonary Hypertension of European Society of Cardiology (ESC) (2009) Guidelines for the diagnosis and treatment of pulmonary hypertension. *Eur Heart J* **30**(20): 2493–537.

National Pulmonary Hypertension centres of the UK and Ireland (2007) Consensus statement on the management of pulmonary hypertension in clinical practice in the UK and Ireland *Heart* : 1–42.

Simmoneau G, Robbins IM, Beghetti M, *et al.* (2009). Updated clinical classification of pulmonary hypertension. *J Am Coll Cardiol* 54: 43–54.

**Chapter 2**

# Pathobiology of pulmonary arterial hypertension

Lan Zhao, Chien-Nien Chen, Zhenguo Zhai
and Martin R Wilkins

---

**Key point**

- Pulmonary arterial hypertension is characterized by
  structural remodelling of pulmonary arterioles and
  arteries.

---

## 2.1 Introduction

Pulmonary arterial hypertension (PAH) has a complex pathobiology.
The hallmark of PAH is a distinctive obliterative remodelling of the
pulmonary vasculature that involves all cell elements of the vessel
wall, including endothelial cells, smooth muscle cells, and fibroblasts, as well as abnormalities in platelets and circulating inflammatory cells. In addition, remodelling stimulates the deposition of
connective tissue matrix components such as collagen, elastin, and
fibronectin. Some molecular mechanisms, such as deficiency of prostacyclin and nitric oxide (NO)/cyclic GMP and increased endothelin,
have been elucidated and translated into therapies for PAH (Archer
et al., 2010). Progress in addressing other mechanisms intrinsic to
PAH pathology will provide insights into new therapeutic targets
(Archer et al., 2010).

## 2.2 The pathology of pulmonary arterial hypertension

### 2.2.1 Pulmonary vasoconstriction and thrombosis

Pulmonary resistance vessels, in contrast to systemic vessels, constrict in response to alveolar hypoxia (<60 mmHg). This is a physiological response designed to maintain perfusion/ventilation (V/Q) matching and systemic oxygenation levels (Von Euler & Liljestrand, 1946). The increase in pulmonary vascular resistance in PAH is pathological and related to endothelial dysfunction. The pulmonary endothelium is a source of vasodilators, specifically prostacyclin and nitric oxide, and vasoconstrictors, such as the endothelins. Endothelial dysfunction is an early feature of the disease and an imbalance favouring vasoconstriction is well documented. Local nitric oxide production and bioavailability is reduced (Girgis et al., 2005), prostacyclin synthase expression is reduced (Tuder et al., 1999) and the ratio of thromboxane to prostacyclin is increased (Christman et al., 1992), and circulating endothelin levels are raised (Allen et al., 1993, Giad et al., 1993). Increased circulating natriuretic peptide levels are unable to address the imbalance. Current therapies are based on restoring prostacyclin (with prostanoids), antagonizing endothelin (by receptor blockade) and enhancing nitric oxide and natriuretic peptide induced signalling (by phosphodiesterase inhibition) (Archer et al., 2010). Reduced expression/activity of voltage-gated potassium channels (KV) in pulmonary smooth muscle cells, resulting in the efflux of potassium and increased intracellular calcium, is another likely contributor to vasoconstriction and restoring activity of these channels is a potential treatment strategy (Weir & Archer, 1995). Endothelial dysfunction also promotes vascular thrombosis and in some patients circulating thrombosis inducing factors, such as antiphospholipid antibodies, play a role (Herve et al., 2001). The release of serotonin and platelet-derived growth factor further aggravate vasoconstriction and stimulate cell proliferation and remodelling (Dempsie & Maclean, 2008).

### 2.2.2 Pulmonary vascular inflammation and remodelling

The histological features of small peripheral pulmonary arteries common to nearly all types of Group 1 PAH include intimal proliferation, medial thickening due to smooth muscle cell hyperplasia and hypertrophy and increased deposition of extracellular matrix (Tuder et al., 2007). The role of inflammatory cells and progenitor cells in structural remodelling is increasingly recognized (Hassoun et al., 2009) (Figure 2.1). The resultant proliferative vascular lesion has drawn parallels with dysregulated cell growth in cancer (Rai et al., 2008).

## Fig 2.1 Summary of the complexed pathobiology of pulmonary arterial hypertension (PAH)

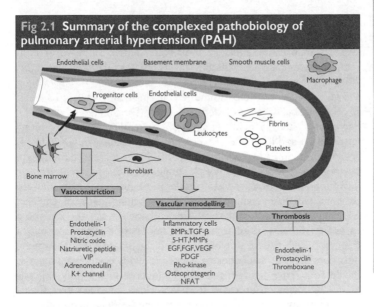

### 2.2.3 Endothelial cells

In addition to disrupting normal vasoconstrictor-vasodilator homeostasis, the injury to endothelial cells, whatever that may be, is believed to cause cell death and the emergence of apoptosis-resistant endothelial cells which then proliferate. The complex plexiform lesions that are found in many PAH patients in the late stages of the disease may comprise an endothelial cell population that is monoclonal in origin (Lee *et al.*, 1998).

### 2.2.4 Smooth muscle cells and fibroblasts

Endothelial cell death exposes unopposed the underlying pulmonary vascular smooth muscle cells to factors from which they would normally be 'protected'. These cells are stimulated to undergo both hypertrophy and hyperplasia and resist apoptosis. This pattern of media thickening results the extension of smooth muscle into distal small peripheral, normally nonmuscular, pulmonary arteries within the respiratory acinus (Meyrick *et al.*, 1980, Tuder *et al.*, 2007, Hassoun *et al.*, 2009, Morrell *et al.*, 2009). Extracellular matrix such as collagen, elastin, fibronectin and tenascin-C contributes to the thickening of pulmonary vascular media and regulate smooth muscle cell growth (Rabinovitch, 2001). In pulmonary precapillary vessels, differentiation of pericytes and intermediate cells into myofibroblasts causes muscularization of partially or non-muscularized small vessels and induces changes in contractile and synthetic properties. Adventitial fibroblasts undergo hyperplasia and markedly increase collagen production, resulting in dramatic increases in adventitial thickness and impaired arterial distensibility (Stenmark *et al.*, 2002).

### 2.2.5 **Inflammatory cells**

Inflammatory cells and activated platelets appear to predominate in later stages of PAH, although their role—either causative or consequential to PAH—is still unclear (Taraseviciene-Stewart et al., 2007, Hassoun et al., 2009). The plexiform lesions in PAH have been shown to be infiltrated by immune cells, including activated T cells, B cells, macrophages and dentritic cells (Dorfmuller et al., 2003, Perros et al., 2007, Sanchez et al., 2007). Several cytokines (e.g. interleukin (IL)-1 and IL-6) and chemokines (e.g. fractalkine, CX3CL113) are increased in PAH (Dorfmuller et al., 2003). Increased monocyte chemoattractant protein, MCP-1, stimulates monocyte/macrophage migration and smooth muscle proliferation. Recent studies indicate patients with PAH exhibit increased circulating levels of CD34+/CD25high (so-called regulatory) T cells (Ulrich et al., 2008). In some cases the stimulus to inflammation is understood in the context of the associated disease, for example, collagen vascular autoimmune disorders such as scleroderma, systemic lupus erythematosus and mixed connective tissue disease and infection, such as HIV (Nicolls et al., 2005). In other cases it is less clear, although endothelial dysfunction can result in increased cytokine production.

### 2.2.6 **Progenitor cells**

Circulating endothelial progenitor cells have been reported to be either reduced (Fadini et al., 2007, Diller et al., 2008, Junhui et al., 2008) or increased (Asosingh et al., 2008, Toshner et al., 2009) in numbers in idiopathic PAH compared with healthy controls. The discrepancy lies with the cell markers used to identify this cell population (Diller et al., 2008, Diller et al., 2010) which have not been standardized. Endothelial progenitor cells have been identified in the vascular lesions of PAH (Toshner et al., 2009). It is not clear whether these cells are involved in the repair or pathogenesis of the vascular lesions. These cells will carry the same germline (and in some cases somatic) gene perturbations that are found in the vascular lesions themselves. This has not diminished interest in using infusions of autologous cells as a treatment, in some cases transfected with a gene (e.g. nitric oxide synthase) to facilitate repair (Wang et al., 2007).

### 2.2.7 **Right ventricular hypertrophy**

The right ventricle (RV) hypertrophies to compensate the increased workload but RV function often worsens over the time (Voelkel et al., 2006). The morbidity and mortality of PH is closely associated with RV haemodynamic function. An increase in wall stress not only increases myocardial oxygen demand but also impedes myocardial perfusion through a reduction in coronary blood flow to the myocardium, which can induce RV ischemia, both acutely and chronically. In addition to myocyte hypertrophy, fibroblast proliferation and fibrosis can adversely affect myocardial performance. Strategies that preserve RV function may have significant impact on prognosis in the disease. This is receiving more attention. The recent documentation of increased expression of phosphodiesterase (PDE) type 5 in hypertrophied myocardium of patients with PAH (Nagendran et al., 2007) suggest one potential target but this has to be balanced against the adverse experience of PDE3 inhibitors in left ventricular failure.

## 2.3 The molecular mechanisms of pulmonary arterial hypertension

Multiple factors, both genetic and acquired, choreograph the development of PAH.

### 2.3.1 Genomic insights into PAH

#### 2.3.1.1 Bone morphorgenetic protein receptor type 2

Mutations in the gene encoding for bone morphorgenetic protein (BMP) receptor type 2 (BMPR2), a member of the transforming growth factor (TGF-β) receptor superfamily, are found in 60% of heritable PAH and 10–30% of sporadic idiopathic PAH cases (Newman et al., 2008). BMPR2 expression is documented in PAH plexiform lesions, predominantly in the pulmonary endothelium, medial smooth muscle cells and macrophages (Atkinson et al., 2002, Newman et al., 2008). It functions as a receptor with serine/threonine kinase activity and activates a complex range of intracellular signallings such as Smad, LIM kinase, p38/MAP kinase/ERK/JNK, and the c-Src pathway. The gene location of BMPR2 mutations in PAH vary but all predict a reduction in BMPR2 function (Atkinson et al., 2002, Newman et al., 2008). In pulmonary arterial endothelial cells, loss of BMPR2 induced by RNA interference increases susceptibility to apoptosis (Teichert-Kuliszewska et al., 2006), which may contribute to rarefaction of the precapillary vasculature. It must be noted that mice with BMPR2 haploinsufficiency (Beppu et al., 2004) or with dominant-negative BMPR2 mutations (West et al., 2004) exhibit relatively unimpressive structural remodelling. This observation together with the fact there are people with BMPR2 mutations who do not have PAH suggests that BMPR2 mutations predispose to PAH, but a 'second hit' is required to express the disease. The nature of this second hit is still an enigma. Other genetic perturbations are under investigation, including polymorphisms of the serotonin transporter. Other BMP and TGF-β receptor family members, such as activin-like kinase type 1 (ALK1) and endoglin that are mutated in hereditary hemorrhagic telangiectasia, have been reported in patients with PAH (Trembath et al., 2001, Trembath & Harrison, 2003).

At the very least, the discovery of an association between PAH and mutations in BMPR2 has drawn attention to the TGF-β signalling pathway as a therapeutic target. Restoring BMPR2 function is a challenge and may not be sufficient. Gene therapy with BMPR2 (McMurtry et al., 2007) did not appear to be sufficient to reverse monocrotaline-induced pulmonary hypertension. As BMPs and TGF-β have opposing actions, a simple model of impaired BMPR2 function suggests unopposed TGF-β activity may be important in the structural remodelling of PAH. In support of this, recent data indicates that ALK5/TGF-β inhibition prevents pulmonary artery smooth muscle cell migration and attenuated the development and progression of PAH in monocrotaline rat model (Long et al., 2009).

### 2.3.1.2 Serotonin and serotonin transporter

Serotonin (5-HT) was first linked to PAH through its association with anorexigen-induced high risk of PAH (Abenhaim et al., 1996). These drugs increase 5-HT availability. 5-HT directly induces smooth muscle hyperplasia after uptake via the cell-surface 5-HT transporter, 5-HTT 11. Pulmonary vascular smooth muscle cells from idiopathic PAH patients show increased 5-HTT expression and undergo enhanced cell proliferation when treated by 5-HT compared to vascular smooth muscle cells from healthy controls (Eddahibi et al., 2001). These findings are supported by the report that mice deficient in 5-HTT or 5-HT-2B, a serotonin receptor, are protected against hypoxia or hypoxia combined with anorexigen dexfenfluamine induced PH (Morecroft et al., 2007, Dempsie et al., 2008). It is also interesting to note that increased serotonin levels enhance normoxic and hypoxic PAP and pulmonary vascular remodelling in BMPR2 heterozygous mouse (Long et al., 2006)

A polymorphism of the 5-HTT gene promoter, the long (L) variant, is associated with increased expression of the transporter and enhanced smooth muscle cell proliferation. The prevalence of this variant is reported to be 65% in idiopathic PAH compared with 27% in the control group (Eddahibi et al., 2001), suggesting that the polymorphysm confers susceptibility to PAH. However this has not been confirmed in larger association studies (Machado et al., 2006).

### 2.3.2 Vasoactive factors influencing pulmonary vascular tone

### 2.3.2.1 Endothelin-1

ET-1 is expressed in pulmonary endothelial cells and acts both as a potent pulmonary arterial vasoconstrictor and mitogen (Hassoun et al., 1992, Stelzner et al., 1992). Increased lung and plasma ET-1 levels are well documented in PAH patients (Allen et al., 1993, Giaid et al., 1993). Binding to the endothelin receptors, A (ETA) and B (ETB), on vascular smooth muscle cells induces an increase in intracellular calcium, along with activation of protein kinase C, mitogen-activated protein kinase and the early growth response genes c-fos and c-jun (Meyrick *et al.*, 1980, Hassoun *et al.*, 2009, Morrell *et al.*, 2009). Binding to the ETB on endothelial cells results in increased nitric oxide and prostacyclin production. Endothelial dysfunction along with a higher prevalence of the ETA receptor in pulmonary resistance arteries suggests that ETA receptor-mediated activity predominates in PAH. Endothelin receptor antagonists, such as bosentan, sitaxentan and ambrisentan, improve pulmonary hae-modynamics, exercise capacity and symptoms (Rubin *et al.*, 2002, Barst *et al.*, 2004, Galie *et al.*, 2008).

### 2.3.2.2 Prostacyclin

Prostacyclin synthase expression is reduced in small and medium-sized pulmonary arteries of lungs from patients with PAH (Tuder *et al.*, 1999) and thromboxane A2 (TXA2) production is favoured (Christman *et al.*, 1992). Prostacyclin activates cyclic adenosine monophosphate (cAMP)-dependent pathways and acts as a vasodi-lator, an antiproliferative agent for vascular smooth muscle (Clapp *et al.*, 2002), and an inhibitor of platelet activation and aggregation. In contrast, TXA2 promotes vasoconstriction and activates platelets (Vanhoutte, 2009). Epoprostenol therapy prolongs survival in idiopathic PAH (McLaughlin *et al.*, 2002). Attempts to antagonize TXA2 have been less successful to date.

### 2.3.2.3 Nitric oxide

Nitric oxide is a potent pulmonary arterial vasodilator as well as a direct inhibitor of platelet activation and vascular smooth muscle cell proliferation. Endothelial nitric oxide synthase (eNOS) is regulated by a multitude of vasoactive factors and physiologic stimuli including hypoxia, inflammation, and oxidative stress. PAH patients have low nitric oxide levels in exhaled breath (Girgis *et al.*, 2005) and decreased eNOS expression in lung tissue (Giaid *et al.*, 1995). Correspondingly, mice deficient in eNOS are more susceptible to developing pulmonary hypertension in response to hypoxia, whereas pulmonary gene transfer of eNOS is partially protective (Champion *et al.*, 2002). Mice deficient in tetrahydrobiopterin (BH4), a cofactor for eNOS, selectively develop a pulmonary hypertension phenotype (Khoo *et al.*, 2005). Both inhaled nitric oxide and orally administered PDE5 inhibitors, which act to increase nitric oxide-mediated cGMP signaling, have emerged as therapeutic strategies in pulmonary hypertension (Giaid & Saleh, 1995, Germann *et al.*, 2005, Wilkins *et al.*, 2005). Direct small molecule (e.g. riociguat) stimulation of soluble guanylate cyclase is under investigation as a potential treatment for PAH (Grimminger *et al.*, 2009).

### 2.3.2.4 Natriuretic peptide

Atrial natriuretic peptide (ANP) and B-type natriuretic peptide (BNP) are cardiac hormones with potent diuretic, vascular relaxant, and antiproliferative properties. They act on a membrane-bound receptor that activates particulate guanylate cyclase and promotes cGMP synthesis (Leitman et al., 1988). They inhibit ET-1 synthesis and ET receptor expression (Davie et al., 2002). Studies in mice with targeted disruption of the ANP gene or its receptor suggests ANP protects against the development of pulmonary hypertension and RV hypertrophy (Klinger et al., 1999, Zhao et al., 2003). Circulating levels of BNP are elevated on PAH and correlate with pulmonary arterial pressure and pulmonary vascular resistance, predicting survival (Casserly & Klinger, 2009). Inhibition of neutral endopeptidase, the enzyme responsible of metabolism of natriuretic peptides, in combination with PDE5 inhibition, which augments cyclic GMP signalling, offer a novel approach to the treatment of PAH (Klinger et al., 1999, Baliga et al., 2008).

### 2.3.2.5 Vasoactive intestinal peptide
Vasoactive intestinal peptide (VIP) is a 28 amino-acid peptide which belongs to the glucagon-growth hormone–releasing factor secretion superfamily. VIP deficient mice develop moderate severe PH in normoxia (Said et al., 2007, Hamidi et al., 2008). Intravenous VIP improved tissue oxygenation in a neonatal PAH piglet model and demonstrated selective pulmonary vasodilatory effects (Haydar et al., 2007). In PAH patients, VIP inhalation induces acute but selective pulmonary vasodilation, reduces pulmonary vascular resistance i.e. RV workload (Leuchte et al., 2008). Data on the effect of chronic administration to patients are waited.

### 2.3.2.6 Adrenomedullin
Circulating levels of adrenomedullin (AM), a vasodilator peptide are elevated in PAH patients and correlate with haemodynamic severity of the disease (Zhao et al., 1996, Nishida et al., 2008). AM acts via the calcitonin receptor-like receptor and receptor activity-modifying proteins-2 and -3 (McLatchie et al., 1998) and through several signalling pathways such as cAMP, nitric oxide-cGMP and PI3K/Akt (Kato et al., 2005). Intravenous AM reduces both pulmonary and systemic blood pressure but inhalation therapy offers the potential of pulmonary vascular selectivity (Nagaya et al., 2000, Nagaya et al., 2004, Qi et al., 2007).

### 2.3.3 Potassium channels and mitochondrial metabolism

### 2.3.3.1 Potassium channels
Voltage-dependent potassium (Kv) channel activity is reduced by a number of stimuli that promote PAH, including hypoxia (Weir et al., 2006, Sommer et al., 2008) and fenfluramine derivatives (Weir et al., 1998, Michelakis & Weir, 2001). Expression and

activity of Kv1.5 channels are downregulated in pulmonary vascular smooth muscle cells from PAH patients. Reduced expression of Kv channels favors an influx of intracellular calcium and initiates a number of intracellular signalling cascades promoting vasoconstriction and proliferation and inhibiting apoptosis. Increased expression of Kv channels appears necessary for the apoptosis associated with the actions of BMP2 and dichloroacetate. Gene transfer of Kv channels have been used as an experimental strategy in animal models to prevent and reverse pulmonary hypertension (Pozeg et al., 2003).

### 2.3.3.2 Dichloroacetate

Proliferating cells appear to share a common switch in cellular metabolism, deriving energy from glycolysis rather than oxidative phosphorylation (Warburg effect) (Bonnet et al., 2007, Xu et al., 2007, Fijalkowska et al., 2010). This switch in metabolism is less efficient but confers a proliferative advantage to cells accompanied by resistance to apoptosis. The generic drug, dichloroacetate (DCA), is an orally available small molecule that inhibits pyruvate dehydrogenase kinase, increases the flux of pyruvate into the mitochondria, and promotes glucose oxidation over glycolysis. Early data from oncology studies suggests this renders proliferating cells more susceptible to glycolysis and attenuates tumour growth. DCA activates mitochondria-dependent apoptosis, reverses vascular remodelling, normalizes haemodynamics, attenuates RV hypertrophy and improves survival in several rat models of pulmonary hypertension (Bonnet et al., 2006, Guignabert et al., 2006, Michelakis et al., 2002).

### 2.3.4 **Proliferation and apoptosis mediators**

### 2.3.4.1 Platelet-derived growth factor

Platelet-derived growth factor (PDGF), acting via its receptor tyrosine kinase, has been implicated in smooth muscle cell recruitment and endothelial cell proliferation and dysfunction (Barst, 2005). PDGF receptors are upregulated in lambs with chronic intrauterine pulmonary hypertension (Balasubramaniam et al., 2003) and lung tissue isolates from PAH patients show significant increase in PDGF receptor expression (Humbert et al., 1998). The PDGF receptor antagonist, imatinib, has been shown to inhibit proliferation and migration of pulmonary vascular smooth muscle cells (Perros et al., 2008) and have beneficial effects in both hypoxia and monocrotaline models of pulmonary hypertension (Schermuly et al., 2005). Initial case studies show promise from imatinib as a treatment for PAH and further studies are in progress (Ghofrani et al., 2005, Patterson et al., 2006, Souza et al., 2006).

### 2.3.4.2 Vascular endothelial growth factor (VEGF)

VEGF (VEGF-A), expressed abundantly in the lungs, supports pulmonary endothelial cell survival (Voelkel et al., 2006). VEGF ligand binding to its main receptor, VEGFR-2 tyrosine kinase, results in increased expression of eNOS and increased prostacyclin production. Blockade of VEGFR-2 in newborn rats by the tyrosine kinase inhibitor SU-5416 results in pulmonary hypertension with RV hypertrophy (Taraseviciene-Stewart et al., 2002). In combination with chronic hypoxia, SU-5416 induces endothelial cell apoptosis followed by the emergence of endothelial cells resistant to apoptosis and severe pulmonary hypertension associated with precapillary occlusion (Taraseviciene-Stewart et al., 2001). In PAH, VEGF expression is increased in pulmonary vasculature, especially in plexiform lesions. Overexpression of VEGF by adenovirus-mediated gene transfer attenuates PAH and RV hypertrophy in rats induced by chronic hypoxia (Partovian et al., 2000). Treatment with VEGF reduced the severity of pulmonary hypertension in fetal sheep with partial ligation of the ductus arteriosus (Grover et al., 2005), and VEGF gene transfer attenuated pulmonary hypertension in monocrotaline rats (Campbell et al., 2001). VEGF-B resembles VEGF-A in that its overexpression in the lung attenuates experimental pulmonary hypertension, but its expression is not regulated by hypoxia or cytokines and it does not stimulate eNOS expression or increase vascular permeability (Louzier et al., 2003).

### 2.3.4.3 Rho-kinase

The Rho/Rho-associated kinase (Rho-kinase) system regulates a variety of cellular functions relevant to structural remodelling in PAH, including migration, proliferation and apoptosis (Oka et al., 2008, Wojciak-Stothard, 2008). cAMP- and cGMP-dependent protein kinases (PKA and PKG) have a key role in regulating Rho activation and expression in vascular smooth muscle cells (Sauzeau et al., 2000, Sauzeau et al., 2003). RhoA and its downstream mediator Rho-kinase have become attractive targets for the treatment of PAH (Oka et al., 2008). Rho-kinase inhibitors, such as fasudil, exhibit acute vasodilator effects in patients with PAH (Fukumoto et al., 2005) and inhibit the development of pulmonary hypertension in experimental models (Louzier et al., 2003).

### 2.3.4.4 Osteoprotegerin (OPG)

OPG, a member of the tumour necrosis factor receptor superfamily, is a secreted basic glycoprotein (Yamaguchi et al., 1998). OPG is expressed and secreted by a variety of tissues, including the heart and lung (Simonet et al., 1997). OPG functions as a secreted decoy receptor, competing either with receptor activator of nuclear factor-B (RANK) for the binding of RANK ligand (RANKL) to regulate osteoclast differentiation and activation or with tumour necrosis factor-related apoptosis-inducing ligand (TRAIL), preventing binding to membrane-associated death receptors (DR4 and DR5) to trigger apoptosis of multiple cell types (Emery et al., 1998). Abnormalities in BMP, 5-HT, and inflammatory signalling result in heightened expression of OPG in pulmonary vascular smooth muscle cells. Additionally, OPG increases pulmonary vascular smooth muscle cell proliferation and migration (Lawrie et al., 2008). Immunohistochemistry of human PAH lesions has demonstrated increased OPG expression, and circulating OPG levels are increased in idiopathic PAH and PAH associated with congenital systemic-to-pulmonary shunts (Brun et al., 2009).

### 2.3.4.5 Nuclear factor of activated T cells

NFAT, a transcription factor that regulates T cell activation, cardiac development/hypertrophy, and vascular remodelling, is activated in PAH in vitro and in vivo (Bonnet et al., 2007). NFAT is known to regulate the expression Kv1.5 and bcl-2. Bcl-2 is increased in human PAH and inhibits apoptosis by interacting with the mitochondrial membrane. Inhibition of NFAT reverses the PAH phenotype (upregulating Kv1.5, downregulating bcl-2, and depolarizing mitochondria), induces remodelled vessel wall apoptosis, and attenuates pulmonary hypertension in the rat. Targeting NFAT pharmacologically improves RV contractility by modulating chamber-specific dynamic changes in mitochondrial membrane potential during right ventricular hypertrophy (Nagendran et al., 2008).

## 2.4 **Conclusion**

The pathobiology of PAH is unravelling slowly and each new insight suggests a novel drug target or therapeutic strategy. The challenge now is to draw this together and identify the nodal points where intervention is likely to have the greatest impact. An ideal therapy is one that is selective for the pulmonary vascular bed, reverses established vascular remodelling and is well tolerated. There is now considerable interest from pharmaceutical companies in developing better treatments. There will not be one single treatment. We need an armoury of treatments from which to select the best for each patient according to their personal pathology.

# References

Abenhaim L, Moride Y, Brenot F et al. (1996) Appetite-suppressant drugs and the risk of primary pulmonary hypertension. International Primary Pulmonary Hypertension Study Group. N Engl J Med **335**(9): 609–16.

Ali O, Wharton J, Gibbs JS, Howard L, Wilkins MR (2007) Emerging therapies for pulmonary arterial hypertension. *Expert Opin Investig Drugs* **16**(6): 803–18.

Allen SW, Chatfield BA, Koppenhafer SA, Schaffer MS, Wolfe RR, Abman SH (1993) Circulating immunoreactive endothelin-1 in children with pulmonary hypertension. Association with acute hypoxic pulmonary vasoreactivity. *Am Rev Respir Dis* **148**(2): 519–22.

Archer SL, Weir EK, Wilkins MR (2010) Basic science of pulmonary hypertension for clinicians: New concepts and experimental therapies. *Circulation* **121**(18): 2045–66.

Asosingh K, Aldred MA, Vasanji A et al. (2008) Circulating angiogenic precursors in idiopathic pulmonary arterial hypertension. *Am J Pathol* **172**(3): 615–27.

Atkinson C, Stewart S, Upton PD et al. (2002) Primary pulmonary hypertension is associated with reduced pulmonary vascular expression of type II bone morphogenetic protein receptor. *Circulation* **105**(14): 1672–8.

Balasubramaniam V, Le Cras TD, Ivy DD, Grover TR, Kinsella JP, Abman SH (2003) Role of platelet-derived growth factor in vascular remodeling during pulmonary hypertension in the ovine fetus. *Am J Physiol Lung Cell Mol Physiol* **284**(5): L826–L833.

Baliga RS, Zhao L, Madhani M et al. (2008) Synergy between natriuretic peptides and phosphodiesterase 5 inhibitors ameliorates pulmonary arterial hypertension. *Am J Respir Crit Care Med* **178**(8): 861–9.

Barst RJ, Langleben D, Frost A et al. (2004) Sitaxentan therapy for pulmonary arterial hypertension. *Am J Respir Crit Care Med* **169**(4): 441–7.

Barst RJ (2005) PDGF signaling in pulmonary arterial hypertension. *J Clin Invest* **115**(10): 2691–4.

Beppu H, Ichinose F, Kawai N et al. (2004) BMPR-II heterozygous mice have mild pulmonary hypertension and an impaired pulmonary vascular remodeling response to prolonged hypoxia. *Am J Physiol Lung Cell Mol Physiol* **287**(6): L1241–L1247.

Bonnet S, Michelakis ED, Porter CJ et al. (2006) An abnormal mitochondrial-hypoxia inducible factor-1alpha-Kv channel pathway disrupts oxygen sensing and triggers pulmonary arterial hypertension in fawn hooded rats: similarities to human pulmonary arterial hypertension. *Circulation* **113**(22): 2630–41.

Bonnet S, Archer SL, Ialunis-Turner J et al. (2007a) A mitochondria-K+ channel axis is suppressed in cancer and its normalization promotes apoptosis and inhibits cancer growth. *Cancer Cell* **11**(1): 37–51.

Bonnet S, Rochefort G, Sutendra G et al. (2007b) The nuclear factor of activated T cells in pulmonary arterial hypertension can be therapeutically targeted. *Proc Natl Acad Sci U S A* **104**(27): 11418–23.

Brun H, Holmstrom H, Thaulow E et al. (2009) Patients with pulmonary hypertension related to congenital systemic-to-pulmonary shunts are characterized by inflammation involving endothelial cell activation and platelet-mediated inflammation. *Congenit Heart Dis* **4**(3): 153–9.

Campbell AI, Zhao Y, Sandhu R, Stewart DJ (2001) Cell-based gene transfer of vascular endothelial growth factor attenuates monocrotaline-induced pulmonary hypertension. *Circulation* **104**(18): 2242–8.

Casserly B, Klinger JR (2009) Brain natriuretic peptide in pulmonary arterial hypertension: biomarker and potential therapeutic agent. *Drug Des Devel Ther* **3**: 269–87.

Champion HC, Bivalacqua TJ, Greenberg SS, Giles TD, Hyman AL, Kadowitz PJ (2002) Adenoviral gene transfer of endothelial nitric-oxide synthase (eNOS) partially restores normal pulmonary arterial pressure in eNOS-deficient mice. *Proc Natl Acad Sci U S A* **99**(20): 13248–53.

Christman BW, McPherson CD, Newman JH et al. (1992) An imbalance between the excretion of thromboxane and prostacyclin metabolites in pulmonary hypertension. *N Engl J Med* **327**(2): 70–5.

Clapp LH, Finney P, Turcato S, Tran S, Rubin LJ, Tinker A (2002) Differential effects of stable prostacyclin analogs on smooth muscle proliferation and cyclic AMP generation in human pulmonary artery. *Am J Respir Cell Mol Biol* **26**(2): 194–201.

Davie N, Haleen SJ, Upton PD et al. (2002) ET(A) and ET(B) receptors modulate the proliferation of human pulmonary artery smooth muscle cells. *Am J Respir Crit Care Med* **165**(3): 398–405.

Dempsie Y, Maclean MR (2008) Pulmonary hypertension: therapeutic targets within the serotonin system. *Br J Pharmacol* **155**(4): 455–62.

Dempsie Y, Morecroft I, Welsh DJ et al. (2008) Converging evidence in support of the serotonin hypothesis of dexfenfluramine-induced pulmonary hypertension with novel transgenic mice. *Circulation* **117**(22): 2928–37.

Diller GP, van ES, Okonko DO et al. (2008) Circulating endothelial progenitor cells in patients with Eisenmenger syndrome and idiopathic pulmonary arterial hypertension. *Circulation* **117**(23): 3020–30.

Diller GP, Thum T, Wilkins MR, Wharton J (2010) Ehdothelial progenitor cells in pulmonary arterial hypertension. *Trends in Caridovascular Medicine.* In press.

Dorfmuller P, Perros F, Balabanian K, Humbert M (2003) Inflammation in pulmonary arterial hypertension. *Eur Respir J* **22**(2): 358–63.

Eddahibi S, Humbert M, Fadel E et al. (2001) Serotonin transporter overexpression is responsible for pulmonary artery smooth muscle hyperplasia in primary pulmonary hypertension. *J Clin Invest* **108**(8): 1141–50.

Emery JG, McDonnell P, Burke MB et al. (1998) Osteoprotegerin is a receptor for the cytotoxic ligand TRAIL. *J Biol Chem* **273**(23): 14363–7.

Fadini GP, Schiavon M, Rea F, Avogaro A, Agostini C (2007) Depletion of endothelial progenitor cells may link pulmonary fibrosis and pulmonary hypertension. *Am J Respir Crit Care Med* **176**(7): 724–5.

Fijalkowska I, Xu W, Comhair SA et al. (2010) Hypoxia inducible-factor1alpha regulates the metabolic shift of pulmonary hypertensive endothelial cells. *Am J Pathol* **176**(3): 1130–8.

Fukumoto Y, Matoba T, Ito A et al. (2005) Acute vasodilator effects of a Rho-kinase inhibitor, fasudil, in patients with severe pulmonary hypertension. *Heart* **91**(3): 391–2.

Galie N, Olschewski H, Oudiz RJ et al. (2008) Ambrisentan for the treatment of pulmonary arterial hypertension: results of the ambrisentan in pulmonary arterial hypertension, randomized, double-blind, placebo-controlled, multicenter, efficacy (ARIES) study 1 and 2. *Circulation* **117**(23): 3010–9.

Germann P, Braschi A, Della RG et al. (2005) Inhaled nitric oxide therapy in adults: European expert recommendations. *Intensive Care Med* June 23.

Ghofrani HA, Seeger W, Grimminger F (2005) Imatinib for the treatment of pulmonary arterial hypertension. *N Engl J Med* **353**(13): 1412–3.

Giaid A, Yanagisawa M, Langleben D et al. (1993) Expression of endothelin-1 in the lungs of patients with pulmonary hypertension. *N Engl J Med* **328**(24): 1732–9.

Giaid A, Saleh D (1995) Reduced expression of endothelial nitric oxide synthase in the lungs of patients with pulmonary hypertension. *N Engl J Med* **333**(4): 214–21.

Girgis RE, Champion HC, Diette GB, Johns RA, Permutt S, Sylvester JT (2005) Decreased exhaled nitric oxide in pulmonary arterial hypertension: response to bosentan therapy. *Am J Respir Crit Care Med* **172**(3): 352-7.

Grimminger F, Weimann G, Frey R et al. (2009) First acute haemodynamic study of soluble guanylate cyclase stimulator riociguat in pulmonary hypertension. *Eur Respir J* **33**(4): 785–92.

Grover TR, Parker TA, Abman SH (2005) Vascular endothelial growth factor improves pulmonary vascular reactivity and structure in an experimental model of chronic pulmonary hypertension in fetal sheep. Chest 2005 December;128(6 Suppl):614S.

Guignabert C, Tu L, Izikki M et al. (2009) Dichloroacetate treatment partially regresses established pulmonary hypertension in mice with SM22alpha-targeted overexpression of the serotonin transporter. *FASEB J* **23**(12): 4135–47.

Hamidi SA, Prabhakar S, Said SI (2008) Enhancement of pulmonary vascular remodelling and inflammatory genes with VIP gene deletion. *Eur Respir J* **31**(1): 135–9.

Hassoun PM, Thappa V, Landman MJ, Fanburg BL (1992) Endothelin 1: mitogenic activity on pulmonary artery smooth muscle cells and release from hypoxic endothelial cells. *Proc Soc Exp Biol Med* **199**(2): 165–70.

Hassoun PM, Mouthon L, Barbera JA et al. (2009) Inflammation, growth factors, and pulmonary vascular remodeling. *J Am Coll Cardiol* **54**(1): S10–S19.

Haydar S, Sarti JF, Grisoni ER (2007) Intravenous vasoactive intestinal polypeptide lowers pulmonary-to-systemic vascular resistance ratio in a neonatal piglet model of pulmonary arterial hypertension. *J Pediatr Surg* **42**(5): 758–64.

Herve P, Humbert M, Sitbon O et al. (2001) Pathobiology of pulmonary hypertension. The role of platelets and thrombosis. *Clin Chest Med* **22**(3): 451–8.

Humbert M, Monti G, Fartoukh M et al. (1998) Platelet-derived growth factor expression in primary pulmonary hypertension: comparison of HIV seropositive and HIV seronegative patients. *Eur Respir J* **11**(3): 554–9.

Junhui Z, Xingxiang W, Guosheng F, Yunpeng S, Furong Z, Junzhu C (2008) Reduced number and activity of circulating endothelial progenitor cells in patients with idiopathic pulmonary arterial hypertension. *Respir Med* **102**(7): 1073–9.

Kato J, Tsuruda T, Kita T, Kitamura K, Eto T (2005) Adrenomedullin: a protective factor for blood vessels. *Arterioscler Thromb Vasc Biol* **25**(12): 2480–7.

Khoo JP, Zhao L, Alp NJ et al. (2005) Pivotal role for endothelial tetrahydro-biopterin in pulmonary hypertension. *Circulation* **111**(16): 2126–33.

Klinger JR, Warburton RR, Pietras LA, Smithies O, Swift R, Hill NS (1999) Genetic disruption of atrial natriuretic peptide causes pulmonary hyperten-sion in normoxic and hypoxic mice. *Am J Physiol* **276**(5 Pt 1): L868–L874.

Lawrie A, Waterman E, Southwood M et al. (2008) Evidence of a role for osteoprotegerin in the pathogenesis of pulmonary arterial hypertension. *Am J Pathol* **172**(1): 256–64.

Lee SD, Shroyer KR, Markham NE, Cool CD, Voelkel NF, Tuder RM (1998) Monoclonal endothelial cell proliferation is present in primary but not secondary pulmonary hypertension. *J Clin Invest* **101**(5): 927–34.

Leitman DC, Andresen JW, Catalano RM, Waldman SA, Tuan JJ, Murad F (1988) Atrial natriuretic peptide binding, cross-linking, and stimulation of cyclic GMP accumulation and particulate guanylate cyclase activity in cultured cells. *J Biol Chem* **263**(8): 3720–8.

Leuchte HH, Baezner C, Baumgartner RA et al. (2008) Inhalation of vaso-active intestinal peptide in pulmonary hypertension. *Eur Respir J* **32**(5): 1289–94.

Loirand G, Guerin P, Pacaud P (2006) Rho kinases in cardiovascular physiology and pathophysiology. *Circ Res* **98**(3): 322–34.

Long L, MacLean MR, Jeffery TK et al. (2006) Serotonin increases susceptibil-ity to pulmonary hypertension in BMPR2-deficient mice. *Circ Res* **98**(6): 818–27.

Long L, Crosby A, Yang X et al. (2009) Altered bone morphogenetic protein and transforming growth factor-beta signaling in rat models of pulmonary hypertension: potential for activin receptor-like kinase-5 inhibition in pre-vention and progression of disease. *Circulation* **119**(4): 566–76.

Louzier V, Raffestin B, Leroux A et al. (2003) Role of VEGF-B in the lung during development of chronic hypoxic pulmonary hypertension. *Am J Physiol Lung Cell Mol Physiol* **284**(6): L926–L937.

Machado RD, Koehler R, Glissmeyer E et al. (2006) Genetic association of the serotonin transporter in pulmonary arterial hypertension. *Am J Respir Crit Care Med* **173**(7): 793–7.

McLatchie LM, Fraser NJ, Main MJ et al. (1998) RAMPs regulate the trans-port and ligand specificity of the calcitonin-receptor-like receptor. *Nature* **393**(6683): 333–9.

McLaughlin VV, Shillington A, Rich S (2002) Survival in primary pulmonary hypertension: the impact of epoprostenol therapy. *Circulation* **106**(12): 1477–82.

McMurtry MS, Moudgil R, Hashimoto K, Bonnet S, Michelakis ED, Archer SL (2007) Overexpression of human bone morphogenetic protein receptor 2 does not ameliorate monocrotaline pulmonary arterial hypertension. *Am J Physiol Lung Cell Mol Physiol* **292**(4): L872–L878.

Meyrick B, Reid L (1980) Hypoxia-induced structural changes in the media and adventitia of the rat hilar pulmonary artery and their regression. *Am J Pathol* **100**(1): 151–78.

Michelakis ED, Weir EK (2001) Anorectic drugs and pulmonary hypertension from the bedside to the bench. *Am J Med Sci* **321**(4): 292–9.

Michelakis ED, McMurtry MS, Wu XC et al. (2002) Dichloroacetate, a metabolic modulator, prevents and reverses chronic hypoxic pulmonary hypertension in rats: role of increased expression and activity of voltage-gated potassium channels. *Circulation* **105**(2): 244–50.

Morecroft I, Dempsie Y, Bader M et al. (2007) Effect of tryptophan hydroxylase 1 deficiency on the development of hypoxia-induced pulmonary hypertension. *Hypertension* **49**(1): 232–6.

Morrell NW, Adnot S, Archer SL et al. (2009) Cellular and molecular basis of pulmonary arterial hypertension. *J Am Coll Cardiol* **54**(1): S20–S31.

Nagaya N, Nishikimi T, Uematsu M et al. (2000) Haemodynamic and hormonal effects of adrenomedullin in patients with pulmonary hypertension. *Heart* **84**(6): 653–8.

Nagaya N, Kyotani S, Uematsu M et al. (2004) Effects of adrenomedullin inhalation on hemodynamics and exercise capacity in patients with idiopathic pulmonary arterial hypertension. *Circulation* **109**(3): 351–6.

Nagendran J, Archer SL, Soliman D et al. (2007) Phosphodiesterase type 5 is highly expressed in the hypertrophied human right ventricle, and acute inhibition of phosphodiesterase type 5 improves contractility. *Circulation* **116**(3): 238–48.

Nagendran J, Gurtu V, Fu DZ et al. (2008) A dynamic and chamber-specific mitochondrial remodeling in right ventricular hypertrophy can be therapeutically targeted. *J Thorac Cardiovasc Surg* **136**(1): 168–78.

Newman JH, Phillips JA, III, Loyd JE (2008) Narrative review: the enigma of pulmonary arterial hypertension: new insights from genetic studies. *Ann Intern Med* **148**(4): 278–83.

Nicolls MR, Taraseviciene-Stewart L, Rai PR, Badesch DB, Voelkel NF (2008) Autoimmunity and pulmonary hypertension: a perspective. *Eur Respir J* **26**(6): 1110–8.

Nishida H, Horio T, Suzuki Y et al. (2008) Plasma adrenomedullin as an independent predictor of future cardiovascular events in high-risk patients: Comparison with C-reactive protein and adiponectin. *Peptides* **29**(4): 599–605.

Oka M, Fagan KA, Jones PL, McMurtry IF (2008) Therapeutic potential of RhoA/Rho kinase inhibitors in pulmonary hypertension. *Br J Pharmacol* **155**(4): 444–54.

Partovian C, Adnot S, Raffestin B et al. (2000) Adenovirus-mediated lung vascular endothelial growth factor overexpression protects against hypoxic pulmonary hypertension in rats. *Am J Respir Cell Mol Biol* **23**(6): 762–71.

Patterson KC, Weissmann A, Ahmadi T, Farber HW (2006) Imatinib mesylate in the treatment of refractory idiopathic pulmonary arterial hypertension. *Ann Intern Med* **145**(2): 152–3.

Perros F, Dorfmuller P, Souza R et al. (2007) Dendritic cell recruitment in lesions of human and experimental pulmonary hypertension. *Eur Respir J* **29**(3): 462–8.

Perros F, Montani D, Dorfmuller P et al. (2008) Platelet-derived growth factor expression and function in idiopathic pulmonary arterial hypertension. *Am J Respir Crit Care Med* **178**(1): 81–8.

Pozeg ZI, Michelakis ED, McMurtry MS *et al.* (2003) In vivo gene transfer of the O2-sensitive potassium channel Kv1.5 reduces pulmonary hypertension and restores hypoxic pulmonary vasoconstriction in chronically hypoxic rats. *Circulation* **107**(15): 2037–44.

Qi JG, Ding YG, Tang CS, Du JB (2007) Chronic administration of adrenomedullin attenuates hypoxic pulmonary vascular structural remodeling and inhibits proadrenomedullin N-terminal 20-peptide production in rats. *Peptides* **28**(4): 910–9.

Rabinovitch M (2001) Pathobiology of pulmonary hypertension. Extracellular matrix. *Clin Chest Med* (3): 433–49, viii.

Rai PR, Cool CD, King JA *et al.* (2008) The cancer paradigm of severe pulmonary arterial hypertension. *Am J Respir Crit Care Med* **178**(6): 558–64.

Rubin LJ, Badesch DB, Barst RJ *et al.* (2002) Bosentan therapy for pulmonary arterial hypertension. *N Engl J Med* **346**(12): 896–903.

Said SI, Hamidi SA, Dickman KG *et al.* (2007) Moderate pulmonary arterial hypertension in male mice lacking the vasoactive intestinal peptide gene. *Circulation* **115**(10): 1260–8.

Sanchez O, Marcos E, Perros F *et al.* (2007) Role of endothelium-derived CC chemokine ligand 2 in idiopathic pulmonary arterial hypertension. *Am J Respir Crit Care Med* **176**(10): 1041–7.

Sauzeau V, Le Jeune H, Cario-Toumaniantz C *et al.* (2000) Cyclic GMP-dependent protein kinase signaling pathway inhibits RhoA-induced Ca2+ sensitization of contraction in vascular smooth muscle. *J Biol Chem* **275**(28): 21722–9.

Sauzeau V, Rolli-Derkinderen M, Marionneau C, Loirand G, Pacaud P (2003) RhoA expression is controlled by nitric oxide through cGMP-dependent protein kinase activation. *J Biol Chem* **278**(11): 9472–80.

Schermuly RT, Dony E, Ghofrani HA *et al.* (2005) Reversal of experimental pulmonary hypertension by PDGF inhibition. *J Clin Invest* **115**(10): 2811–21.

Simonet WS, Lacey DL, Dunstan CR *et al.* (1997) Osteoprotegerin: a novel secreted protein involved in the regulation of bone density. *Cell* **89**(2): 309–19.

Sommer N, Dietrich A, Schermuly RT *et al.* (2008) Regulation of hypoxic pulmonary vasoconstriction: basic mechanisms. *Eur Respir J* **32**(6): 1639–51.

Souza R, Sitbon O, Parent F, Simonneau G, Humbert M (2006) Long term imatinib treatment in pulmonary arterial hypertension. *Thorax* **61**(8): 736.

Stelzner TJ, O'Brien RF, Yanagisawa M *et al.* (1992) Increased lung endothelin-1 production in rats with idiopathic pulmonary hypertension. *Am J Physiol* **262**(5 Pt 1): L614–L620.

Stenmark KR, Gerasimovskaya E, Nemenoff RA, Das M (2002) Hypoxic activation of adventitial fibroblasts: role in vascular remodeling. *Chest* **122**(6): 326S–34S.

Taraseviciene-Stewart L, Kasahara Y, Alger L *et al.* (2001) Inhibition of the VEGF receptor 2 combined with chronic hypoxia causes cell death-dependent pulmonary endothelial cell proliferation and severe pulmonary hypertension. *FASEB J* **15**(2): 427–38.

Taraseviciene-Stewart L, Gera L, Hirth P, Voelkel NF, Tuder RM, Stewart JM (2002) A bradykinin antagonist and a caspase inhibitor prevent severe pulmonary hypertension in a rat model. *Can J Physiol Pharmacol* **80**(4): 269–74.

Taraseviciene-Stewart L, Nicolls MR, Kraskauskas D *et al.* (2007) Absence of T cells confers increased pulmonary arterial hypertension and vascular remodeling. *Am J Respir Crit Care Med* **175**(12): 1280–9.

Teichert-Kuliszewska K, Kutryk MJ, Kuliszewski MA *et al.* (2006) Bone morphogenetic protein receptor-2 signaling promotes pulmonary arterial endothelial cell survival: implications for loss-of-function mutations in the pathogenesis of pulmonary hypertension. *Circ Res* **98**(2): 209–17.

Toshner M, Voswinckel R, Southwood M *et al.* (2009) Evidence of dysfunction of endothelial progenitors in pulmonary arterial hypertension. *Am J Respir Crit Care Med* **180**(8): 780–7.

Trembath RC, Thomson JR, Machado RD *et al.* (2001) Clinical and molecular genetic features of pulmonary hypertension in patients with hereditary hemorrhagic telangiectasia. *N Engl J Med* **345**(5): 325–34.

Trembath RC, Harrison R (2003) Insights into the genetic and molecular basis of primary pulmonary hypertension. *Pediatr Res* **53**(6): 883–8.

Tuder RM, Cool CD, Geraci MW *et al.* (1999) Prostacyclin synthase expression is decreased in lungs from patients with severe pulmonary hypertension. *Am J Respir Crit Care Med* **159**(6): 1925–32.

Tuder RM, Marecki JC, Richter A, Fijalkowska I, Flores S (2007) Pathology of pulmonary hypertension. *Clin Chest Med* **28**(1): 23–42, vii.

Ulrich S, Nicolls MR, Taraseviciene L, Speich R, Voelkel N (2008) Increased regulatory and decreased CD8+ cytotoxic T cells in the blood of patients with idiopathic pulmonary arterial hypertension. *Respiration* **75**(3): 272–80.

Vanhoutte PM (2009) COX-1 and vascular disease. *Clin Pharmacol Ther* **86**(2): 212–5.

Voelkel NF, Quaife RA, Leinwand LA *et al.* (2006a) Right ventricular function and failure: report of a National Heart, Lung, and Blood Institute working group on cellular and molecular mechanisms of right heart failure. *Circulation* **114**(17): 1883–91.

Voelkel NF, Vandivier RW, Tuder RM (2006b) Vascular endothelial growth factor in the lung. *Am J Physiol Lung Cell Mol Physiol* **290**(2): L209–L221.

Von Euler US, Liljestrand G (1946) Observations on the pulmonary arterial blood pressure in the cat. *Acta Physiol Scand* **12**: 301–20.

Wang XX, Zhang FR, Shang YP *et al.* (2007) Transplantation of autologous endothelial progenitor cells may be beneficial in patients with idiopathic pulmonary arterial hypertension: a pilot randomized controlled trial. *J Am Coll Cardiol* **49**(14): 1566–71.

Weir EK, Archer SL (1995) The mechanism of acute hypoxic pulmonary vasoconstriction: the tale of two channels. *FASEB J* **9**(2): 183–9.

Weir EK, Reeve HL, Johnson G, Michelakis ED, Nelson DP, Archer SL (1998) A role for potassium channels in smooth muscle cells and platelets in the etiology of primary pulmonary hypertension. *Chest* **114**(3 Suppl): 200S–4S.

Weir EK, Olschewski A (2006) Role of ion channels in acute and chronic responses of the pulmonary vasculature to hypoxia. *Cardiovasc Res* **71**(4): 630–41.

West J, Fagan K, Steudel W *et al.* (2004) Pulmonary hypertension in transgenic mice expressing a dominant-negative BMPRII gene in smooth muscle. *Circ Res* **94**(8): 1109–14.

Wilkins MR, Paul GA, Strange JW *et al.* (2005) Sildenafil versus Endothelin Receptor Antagonist for Pulmonary Hypertension (SERAPH) Study. *Am J Respir Crit Care Med* March 4.

Wojciak-Stothard B (2008) New drug targets for pulmonary hypertension: Rho GTPases in pulmonary vascular remodelling. *Postgrad Med J* **84**(993): 348–53.

Xu W, Koeck T, Lara AR *et al.* (2007) Alterations of cellular bioenergetics in pulmonary artery endothelial cells. *Proc Natl Acad Sci U S A* **104**(4): 1342–7.

Yamaguchi K, Kinosaki M, Goto M *et al.* (1998) Characterization of structural domains of human osteoclastogenesis inhibitory factor. *J Biol Chem* **273**(9): 5117–23.

Zhao L, Brown LA, Owji AA *et al.* (1996) Adrenomedullin activity in chronically hypoxic rat lungs. *Am J Physiol* **271**(2 Pt 2): H622–H629.

Zhao L, Mason NA, Strange JW, Walker H, Wilkins MR (2003) Beneficial effects of phosphodiesterase 5 inhibition in pulmonary hypertension are influenced by natriuretic Peptide activity. *Circulation* **107**(2): 234–7.

## Chapter 3

# Genetics

Rajiv D Machado and Richard C Trembath

| Key points |
|---|
| • BMPR2 is the major genetic cause of PAH |
| • Haploinsufficiency |
| • Incomplete penetrance |
| • Modifier genes |
| • Rare disease alleles. |

## 3.1 Introduction

A heritable basis to pulmonary arterial hypertension (PAH) was initially observed by Dresdale in 1954 (Dresdale et al., 1954). Familial clustering has since been recorded in approximately 10% of the patient population although, due to the complex features of inheritance in PAH, it is widely acknowledged that the proportion of patients with one or more affected relatives is likely to be higher. Indeed, familial PAH has since been reclassified as heritable or HPAH in light of the fact that a germline genetic defect may be transmissible to future generations in as many as a third of all cases (Rich et al., 1987, Simonneau et al., 2009). In the majority of cases, PAH is idiopathic arising spontaneously without familial sharing and without a detectable underlying genetic cause. PAH may occur in association with known risk factors, for example, fenfluramine and dexfenfluramine derived appetite suppressant drugs, or other disorders including thromboembolic disease, connective tissue disease, congenital heart disorders and human immunodeficiency virus (HIV) infection (Runo & Loyd, 2003). The classical features of vasoconstriction and pulmonary arteriole remodelling are observed in all forms of PAH, suggesting a common aetiology although shared disease pathways remain to be fully elucidated.

## 3.2 Clinical and genetic features of PAH

Familial PAH segregates as an autosomal dominant Mendelian trait but with features of complex disease, in particular, markedly reduced penetrance as indicated by asymptomatic obligate carriers and the skipping of entire generations. In all forms of PAH, gender plays a major role as a risk factor with twice as many females affected than males. While PAH may occur at any stage, onset is predominantly in the third decade of life. Notably, the age of disease onset can vary widely both within and between pedigrees (Rich *et al.*, 1987, Loyd *et al.*, 1995, Runo & Loyd, 2003). These features support the concept of a threshold model of disease indicating a requirement for additional genetic and/or environmental factors in disease precipitation (Figure 3.1).

## 3.3 Linkage analysis in familial PAH

The establishment of DNA banks from multi-generational pedigrees, world-wide, in harness with significant developments in genetic mapping and high-throughput genotyping technology, has enabled major advances in the successful linkage of Mendelian disorders to delineated regions of the genome. The utilization of such resources led to the identification of the genetic locus for PAH, on the long arm of chromosome 2q31-33, by two independent research centres.

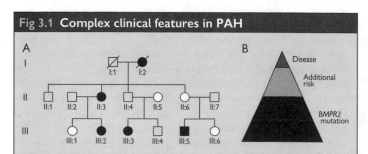

### Fig 3.1 Complex clinical features in PAH

A. Idealized PAH multi-generational pedigree illustrating the characteristic features of PAH including reduced penetrance of the disease allele, as indicated by the absence of manifest disease in the obligate gene carriers II:4 and II:6, and the female preponderance of disease. Affected subjects are indicated by the filled symbols; males and females are indicated by squares and circles, respectively. B. Representation of PAH as a threshold model of disease wherein the black section indicates the risk to patients posed by *BMPR2* mutation. Disease, as indicated by the dark grey apex, is often only precipitated in the presence of additional genetic and/or environmental risk factors, in grey.

Each using linkage analysis with an autosomal dominant model of inheritance, Morse et al. analysed 3 PAH families and Nichols et al. 6 kindreds to isolate minimal linkage intervals of 27 centiMorgans (cM) and 25 cM, with LOD scores of 3.87 and 6.97 respectively (Morse et al., 1997, Nichols et al., 1997).

The cloning of the causative gene was much aided by the construction of a physical map of the region using a combination of YAC, BAC and PAC clones (Machado et al., 2000). The purpose of this map was three-fold: (i) to correct positional ambiguity in the genetic maps; (ii) to determine the physical size of the interval and (iii) to assess the number and position of transcriptional units contained within the minimal region. Subsequent fine-mapping of the extended linkage interval, through the analysis of recombination events occurring in disease haplotypes across all available families, narrowed the interval to 4.8 cM (5.8 Megabases) (Machado et al., 2000). Of the 79 transcripts within the region, those with putative biological relevance to PAH were prioritized for mutation screening by Sanger sequencing. Using this approach, heterozygous germ-line mutations in the gene encoding BMPR-II, a type II bone morphogenetic protein receptor of the TGF-superfamily of cytokines, were identified as the underlying and major genetic defect in familial PAH (Deng et al., 2000, Lane et al., 2000).

## 3.4 Structure and function of BMPR-II

Preceded by a transcriptional start site approximately 1.4 kilobases (kb) upstream of the ATG, the *BMPR2* gene consists of 13 protein coding exons followed by an unusually extended 3 untranslated region (UTR) (Massague, 1998, Aldred et al., 2007, Miyazono et al., 2010). The receptor product comprises 4 major functional domains: an extracellular domain generated by exons 2 and 3; a short transmembrane domain (exon 4); a catalytic serine/threonine kinase domain (exons 5–11); and a cytoplasmic tail (exons 12-13), significantly larger than other receptor species within the TGF-family (Kawabata et al., 1995, Liu et al., 1995). BMPR-II functions by initiating a phosphorylation relay at the cell surface which is ultimately communicated to the nucleus. BMPR-II partners with a specific type I receptor species, which may be BMPR-1A, -1B or ALK1, in a cell-specific manner to efficiently contact extracellular ligand. The close proximity engendered by ligand binding permits the constitutively active BMPR-II to phosphorylate and, thereby, activate the type I receptor which, in turn, phosphorylates specific members of the receptor (R)-Smad family. Stimulated R-Smads 1, 5 and 8 bind Smad 4, common to the entire TGF-family, in the cytosol and shuttle to the nucleus where, in concert with additional transcription factors, they regulate the transcriptional activity of a series of genes. Whilst the Smad system remains the most extensively characterized, the existence of multiple Smad-independent pathways capable of transducing BMP signals has now been established. These include other kinases, for example, p38MAPK and cytoskeletal binding partners such as Tctex-1 and LIMK1. Together, these signalling elements control critical cellular functions including apoptosis, differentiation, proliferation and migration (Massague, 1998, Foletta *et al.*, 2003, Machado *et al.*, 2003, Shi & Massague, 2003, Miyazono *et al.*, 2010).

## 3.5 BMPR2 loss-of-function constitutes the major genetic risk in PAH

Since the seminal studies, in 2000, first identifying deleterious mutations of *BMPR2* in PAH, large cohorts of patients have been analysed across international centres. When taken together, these investigations have allowed for an advanced understanding of the spectrum of mutations in the gene and the molecular mechanism of disease. To date, over 300 private mutations have been detected in patients using technologies to screen for both point mutations and large gene rearrangements (Machado *et al.* 2009). At present, pathogenic defects have been detected in 70% of all familial cases analysed and between 10–40% of subjects without a previously known family history of disease, with no discernible difference in mutation class or distribution (Thomason *et al.*, 2000, Koehler *et al.*, 2004, Morisaki *et al.*, 2004, Aldred *et al.*, 2006). At far lower frequencies, *BMPR2* mutations have been reported in cases where PAH was ascertained in association with other disorders (Figure 3.2) (Humbert *et al.*, 2002, Roberts *et al.*, 2004, Machado *et al.*, 2006, Machado *et al.*, 2009). Approximately 70% of all mutations in familial and idiopathic PAH indicate premature truncation of the transcript by the introduction of early termination codons and are created by a range of mutation types including nonsense (29%), frame-shift (24%), splice-site (9%) and gene rearrangements (6%) (Machado *et al.*, 2009). The terminal *BMPR2* exon 13 is spared from truncating point mutations suggesting that the majority of mutant alleles likely trigger the nonsense-mediated decay (NMD) pathway. NMD studies conducted on patient cell lines and reporter-based *in vitro* systems have both confirmed that these alleles are, indeed, efficiently degraded by the NMD machinery (Aldred *et al.*, 2007, Austin *et al.*, 2009, Hamid *et al.*, 2009). Thus, in the majority of patients, haploinsufficiency is likely to represent the molecular mechanism of disease (Machado *et al.*, 2001, Machado *et al.*, 2009).

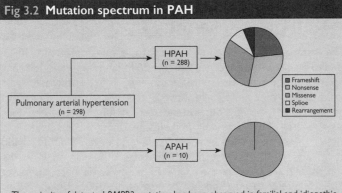

**Fig 3.2 Mutation spectrum in PAH**

The majority of detected *BMPR2* mutation has been observed in familial and idiopathic disease, now classified as HPAH. Ten mutations have been reported in PAH associated with other diseases or risk factors (APAH), namely congenital heart disease, thromboembolic disease and dex/fenfluramine usage. The categories of mutations detected in HPAH and APAH are shown by the pie-charts and described in the boxed key.

## 3.6 **Functional consequences of amino acid substitutions**

Missense mutations in H/IPAH patients are typically confined to exons encoding key functional domains. Ligand binding is contingent upon the structural integrity and folding of the extracellular domain, itself entirely dependent on the formation of five disulphide bonds by 10 cysteine residues encoded by exons 2 and 3 (Greenwald et al., 1999). The critical importance of these amino acids to receptor activity is indicated by the fact that as many as 17 independent mutations, substituting 8 of the 10 cysteine residues, have been recorded in PAH (Machado et al., 2009). Immunofluorescence studies have demonstrated that mutant constructs harbouring these variants are incapable of normal trafficking to the cell surface likely due to major misfolding defects of the mature protein. Cysteine substitutions in the kinase domain result in similar consequences for the receptor; by contrast, non-cysteine substitutions localize correctly but display a much reduced signalling capacity to wild-type when assessed by luciferase assay systems with upstream Smad binding element motifs (Nishihara et al., 2002, Rudarakanchana et al., 2002). Eukaryotic protein kinases are highly conserved across all species and contain residues indispensible to catalytic activity (Hanks & Hunter, 1995). In H/IPAH, mutations within this domain frequently impact upon such residues, for example the arginine at position 491, a site of recurrent mutation which is therefore expected to have a critical impact on receptor function (Machado et al., 2006).

## 3.7 Perturbation of Smad-independent pathways by amino acid substitutions

The vast majority of mutations in the cytoplasmic domain of BMPR-II lead to premature truncation, with only 8 missense mutations having been identified in this region (Machado *et al.*, 2009). Luciferase assays indicate that these amino acid substitutions have no significant effect on the Smad pathway but instead disrupt functional interactions with several BMPR-II binding proteins, amongst them Tctex-1 and LIMK1 (Rudarakanchana *et al.*, 2002, Foletta *et al.*, 2003, Machado *et al.*, 2003). All missense mutations tested thus far result in the constitutive activation of the p38MAPK pathway via mechanisms yet to be fully elucidated (Rudarakanchana *et al.*, 2002, Sankelo *et al.*, 2005). The pertinence of these observations to PAH pathogenesis is unclear and remains under study.

## 3.8 Variants of unknown significance in PAH

At low frequency, *BMPR2* mutations have been observed in PAH associated with other disorders, namely congenital heart disease and thromboembolic disease, and with appetite suppressant usage (Humbert *et al.*, 2002, Roberts *et al.*, 2004, Machado *et al.*, 2009). The mutation spectrum in associated forms of PAH (APAH?) is remarkably distinct to H/IPAH as illustrated by the observation that all identified mutations are unique missense mutations residing in regions of unclear functional significance. Indeed, *in vitro* studies examining the effect of these variants indicate that receptor activity is relatively preserved implying that they may represent low-risk alleles which require additional triggers of large effect size to precipitate disease (Nasim *et al.*, 2008).

## 3.9 Genotype/phenotype correlations in PAH

Correlation of inherited *BMPR2* defects to clinical phenotypes including prognosis, levels of arterial pressure and histopathology in patients have not been observed. In addition, age at disease onset in mutation-positive pedigrees displays wide variability and has been reported to range from 1 to 42 years in a single family (Machado *et al.*, 2001). While broad phenotypic correlations of this nature are not evident, recent studies have demonstrated that a significant number of mutation carriers do not respond to an acute vasodilator challenge. Specifically, Elliott *et al.* observed vasoreactivity in only 3.7%–4% of patients with identified *BMPR2* variants in contrast to 35% of patients without identifiable gene defects Elliott *et al.*, 2006).

These data would suggest that *BMPR2* mutations may have a role in disrupting subtle aspects of pulmonary vascular development and other similar processes equally difficult to quantify.

## 3.10 Recurrent mutation and founder effects in PAH

Approximately half of all mutations identified in independent PAH cases have been observed on multiple occasions, indicating a high incidence of mutation recurrence. The majority (~75%) of these mutations occur at CpG dinucleotide sites implicating methylated cytosine deamination followed by conversion to thymidine as a putative mutational mechanism. Frameshift events resulting from short insertions or deletions typically occur in regions of low sequence complexity, for example mononucleotide repeat elements, suggesting that these mutations may have arisen through replication slippage. Formal investigation into whether this form of mutation is due to founder effects has been limited. However, in the case of three recurrent mutations (p.R332X, p.N861fsX10 and p.R899X), haplotype data generated by genotyping flanking microsatellite markers clearly indicated that the mutations arose independently on distinct genetic backgrounds (Machado *et al.*, 2001). In a nationwide study of PAH in the relatively genetically homogeneous population of Finland, all of the *BMPR2* mutations detected were distinct, once again suggestive of an absence of ancestral mutations (Sankelo *et al.*, 2005). Epidemiological studies remain to be conducted in large patient series, leaving open the possibility that founder effects may yet explain a proportion of recurrent mutation.

37

## 3.11 Rare mutation in members of the TGF-β family underlying PAH

Hereditary haemorrhagic telangiectasia (HHT) is a vascular disorder clinically characterized by the appearance of telangiectasia and widespread arterio-venous malformations (AVMs). In families, HHT segregates as an autosomal dominant trait where the main causal genetic factors are heterozygous mutations of ALK-1 and endoglin, both receptor members of the TGF-family. Of interest, Smad 4 mutations have, on rare occasions, been identified in cases of HHT associated with juvenile polyposis (Abdalla *et al.*, 2005, Prigoda *et al.*, 2006). Infrequently, HHT patients present with PAH identical, clinically and histologically, to the inherited form of the disease. Genotyping of this cohort for *BMPR2*, *ALK1* and *endoglin* revealed that the majority of patients harboured pathogenic mutations of the type I receptor ALK-1. A significant proportion (20%) of the overall

ALK-1 mutation load is associated with the development of PAH; of these, 80% are specific to PAH-HHT. The majority of these mutations lead to amino acid substitutions in the key functional domains of the receptor, namely the GS and kinase domains and the so-called NANDOR box. Thus far, only 4 mutations have been detected in endoglin, all of which lead to premature truncation suggestive of a different mutational mechanism to the ALK-1 defects (Chaouat *et al.*, 2004, Abdalla *et al.*, 2005, Harrison *et al.*, 2005, Mache *et al.*, 2008). A recent study reported ALK-1 mutations in a panel of 9 early-onset PAH cases with no evidence of HHT. Whilst potentially of great interest, it is important to note that the majority of these subjects were extremely young and could go on to develop HHT at a later stage (Fujiwara *et al.*, 2008). The involvement of these receptors in PAH pathogenesis powerfully emphasizes the major role played by TGF-signalling in the maintenance of the pulmonary vasculature.

## 3.12 **Polymorphic variation as risk modifiers in PAH**

The many complex features of PAH, in particular the markedly reduced penetrance, gender bias and variability in age at disease onset within families, suggests that as yet unidentified common genetic variation may play a role in modulating disease development and progression. This hypothesis has been addressed by at least 10 association studies examining common variation in the angiotensin converting enzyme, the serotonin transporter, endoglin, prostacyclin synthase and the potassium channel Kv1.5 (Eddahibi *et al.*, 2001, Aldashev *et al.*, 2002, Abraham *et al.*, 2003, Hoeper *et al.*, 2003, Amano *et al.*, 2004, Koehler *et al.*, 2005, Machado *et al.*, 2006, Willers *et al.*, 2006, Remillard *et al.*, 2007, Wipff *et al.*, 2007). However, all of these studies have been severely compromised by the utilization of case/control cohorts of insufficient magnitude to detect modifying factors of even moderate effect size. This deficiency is well exemplified by the contradictory results reported by different centres of the same analysed variation, in particular the promoter polymorphisms of the serotonin transporter (Eddahibi *et al.*, 2001, Machado *et al.*, 2006). It has become increasingly apparent that significantly larger sample numbers will be required to meaningfully conduct future studies of this nature.

## 3.13 **Animal models of PAH**

To recapitulate the PAH phenotype in an animal model is desirable as it would provide both an important resource of mutant cells for molecular analysis and facilitate studies designed to test potential and novel therapies. Four major murine models have, thus far, been engineered for these purposes. Beppu *et al.* employed a targeted homologous recombination strategy to excise exons 4 and 5 of *BMPR2* in the mouse. Homozygous mutant mice were not viable and displayed wide-ranging developmental defects (Beppu *et al.*, 2000). To gain insight into the role of the gene in later development, Delot *et al.* knocked-out exon 2 of the gene, which left the transcript in-frame, thereby generating a hypomorphic mutant allele. In the homozygous state this mouse died *in utero* but at a later stage, which served to underline the importance of BMPR-II in cardiac development, in particular outflow tract formation (Delot *et al.*, 2003). In both the models described, heterozygotes were viable and broadly phenotypically normal. The likely existence of a critical threshold of BMPR-II activity, below which disease is precipitated, is indicated by two transgenic mouse models over-expressing mutant constructs encoding the disease alleles c.504insT and c.2695C>T (West *et al.*, 2004, West *et al.*, 2008). Although, in nature, these mutations are likely to be lost by NMD these artificial constructs would be capable of producing stable protein capable of acting in a dominant-negative manner by the sequestration of WT receptor in signalling-inactive complexes.

## 3.14 **Future directions**

A better understanding of the critical pathways that intersect with BMPR-II in normal signalling and in disease pathogenesis will be contingent on a combination of genetic and protein-based studies. The identification of rare risk alleles and genetic modifiers of PAH is very clearly in progress as a consequence of international collaborative efforts and the massive advancement of cost-effective genotyping and sequencing technology. These studies in concert with protein-protein interaction investigations aimed at uncovering novel arms of the pathway will continue to provide a launching pad for the development of new therapies.

## References

Abdalla SA, Cymerman U, Rushlow D, Chen N, Stoeber GP, Lemire EG, Letarte M (2005) Novel mutations and polymorphisms in genes causing hereditary hemorrhagic telangiectasia. *Hum Mutat* **25**: 320–1.

Abraham WT, Raynolds MV, Badesch DB *et al.* (2003) Angiotensin-converting enzyme DD genotype in patients with primary pulmonary hypertension: increased frequency and association with preserved haemodynamics. *J Renin Angiotensin Aldosterone Syst* **4**: 27–30.

Aldashev AA, Sarybaev AS, Sydykov AS et al. (2002) Characterization of high-altitude pulmonary hypertension in the Kyrgyz: association with angiotensin-converting enzyme genotype. Am J Respir Crit Care Med **166**: 1396–402.

Aldred MA, Vijayakrishnan J, James V et al. (2006) BMPR2 gene rearrangements account for a significant proportion of mutations in familial and idiopathic pulmonary arterial hypertension. Hum Mutat **27**: 212–3.

Aldred MA, Machado RD, James V, Morrell NW, Trembath RC (2007) Characterization of the BMPR2 5'-untranslated region and a novel mutation in pulmonary hypertension. Am J Respir Crit Care Med **176**: 819–24.

Amano S, Tatsumi K, Tanabe N et al. (2004) Polymorphism of the promoter region of prostacyclin synthase gene in chronic thromboembolic pulmonary hypertension. Respirology **9**: 184–9.

Austin ED, Phillips JA, Cogan JD et al. (2009) Truncating and missense BMPR2 mutations differentially affect the severity of heritable pulmonary arterial hypertension. Respir Res **10**: 87.

Beppu H, Kawabata M, Hamamoto T, Chytil A, Minowa O, Noda T, Miyazono K (2000) BMP type II receptor is required for gastrulation and early development of mouse embryos. Dev Biol **221**: 249–58.

Chaouat A, Coulet F, Favre C, Simonneau G, Weitzenblum E, Soubrier F, Humbert M (2004) Endoglin germline mutation in a patient with hereditary haemorrhagic telangiectasia and dexfenfluramine associated pulmonary arterial hypertension. Thorax **59**: 446–8.

Délot EC, Bahamonde ME, Zhao M, Lyons KM (2003) BMP signaling is required for septation of the outflow tract of the mammalian heart. Development **130**: 209–20.

Deng Z, Morse JH, Slager SL et al. (2000) Familial primary pulmonary hypertension (gene PPH1) is caused by mutations in the bone morphogenetic protein receptor-II gene. Am J Hum Genet **67**: 737–44.

Dresdale DT, Michtom RJ, Schultz M (1954) Recent studies in primary pulmonary hypertension, including pharmacodynamic observations on pulmonary vascular resistance. Bull N Y Acad Med **30**: 195–207.

Eddahibi S, Humbert M, Fadel E et al. (2001) Serotonin transporter overexpression is responsible for pulmonary artery smooth muscle hyperplasia in primary pulmonary hypertension. J Clin Invest **108**: 1141–50.

Elliott CG, Glissmeyer EW, Havlena GT et al. (2006) Relationship of BMPR2 mutations to vasoreactivity in pulmonary arterial hypertension. Circulation **113**: 2509–15.

Foletta VC, Lim MA, Soosairajah J et al. (2003) Direct signaling by the BMP type II receptor via the cytoskeletal regulator LIMK1. J Cell Biol **162**: 1089-98.

Fujiwara M, Yagi H, Matsuoka R et al. (2008) Implications of mutations of activin receptor-like kinase 1 gene (ALK1) in addition to bone morphogenetic protein receptor II gene (BMPR2) in children with pulmonary arterial hypertension. Circ J **72**: 127–33.

Greenwald J, Fischer WH, Vale WW, Choe S (1999) Three-finger toxin fold for the extracellular ligand-binding domain of the type II activin receptor serine kinase. Nat Struct Biol **6**: 18–22.

Hamid R, Cogan JD, Hedges LK, Austin E, Phillips JA, 3rd, Newman JH, Loyd JE (2009) Penetrance of pulmonary arterial hypertension is modulated by the expression of normal BMPR2 allele. *Hum Mutat* **30**: 649–54.

Hanks SK, Hunter T (1995) Protein kinases 6. The eukaryotic protein kinase superfamily: kinase (catalytic) domain structure and classification. *Faseb J* **9**: 576–96.

Harrison RE, Berger R, Haworth SG et al. (2005) Transforming growth factor-beta receptor mutations and pulmonary arterial hypertension in childhood. *Circulation* **111**: 435–41.

Hoeper MM, Tacacs A, Stellmacher U, Lichtinghagen R (2003) Lack of association between angiotensin converting enzyme (ACE) genotype, serum ACE activity, and haemodynamics in patients with primary pulmonary hypertension. *Heart* **89**: 445–6.

Humbert M, Deng Z, Simonneau G et al. (2002) BMPR2 germline mutations in pulmonary hypertension associated with fenfluramine derivatives. *Eur Respir J* **20**: 518–23.

Kawabata M, Chytil A, Moses HL (1995) Cloning of a novel type II serine/threonine kinase receptor through interaction with the type I transforming growth factor-beta receptor. *J Biol Chem* **270**: 5625–30.

Koehler R, Grunig E, Pauciulo MW et al. (2004) Low frequency of BMPR2 mutations in a German cohort of patients with sporadic idiopathic pulmonary arterial hypertension. *J Med Genet* **41**: e127.

Koehler R, Olschewski H, Hoeper M, Janssen B, Grunig E (2005) Serotonin transporter gene polymorphism in a cohort of German patients with idiopathic pulmonary arterial hypertension or chronic thromboembolic pulmonary hypertension. *Chest* **128**: 619S.

Lane KB, Machado RD, Pauciulo MW, Thomson JR, Phillips JA, 3rd, Loyd JE, Nichols WC, Trembath RC (2000) Heterozygous germline mutations in BMPR2, encoding a TGF-beta receptor, cause familial primary pulmonary hypertension. *Nat Genet* **26**: 81–4.

Liu F, Ventura F, Doody J, Massague J (1995) Human type II receptor for bone morphogenic proteins (BMPs): extension of the two-kinase receptor model to the BMPs. *Mol Cell Biol* **15**: 3479–86.

Loyd JE, Butler MG, Foroud TM, Conneally PM, Phillips JA, 3rd, Newman JH (1995) Genetic anticipation and abnormal gender ratio at birth in familial primary pulmonary hypertension. *Am J Respir Crit Care Med* **152**: 93–7.

Machado RD, Pauciulo MW, Fretwell N et al. (2000) A physical and transcript map based upon refinement of the critical interval for PPH1, a gene for familial primary pulmonary hypertension. The International PPH Consortium. *Genomics* **68**: 220–8.

Machado RD, Pauciulo MW, Thomson JR et al. (2001) BMPR2 haploinsufficiency as the inherited molecular mechanism for primary pulmonary hypertension. *Am J Hum Genet* **68**: 92–102.

Machado RD, Rudarakanchana N, Atkinson C, Flanagan JA, Harrison R, Morrell NW, Trembath RC (2003) Functional interaction between BMPR-II and Tctex-1, a light chain of Dynein, is isoform-specific and disrupted by mutations underlying primary pulmonary hypertension. *Hum Mol Genet* **12**: 3277–86.

Machado RD, Aldred MA, James V et al. (2006) Mutations of the TGF-beta type II receptor BMPR2 in pulmonary arterial hypertension. *Hum Mutat* **27**: 121–32.

Machado RD, Koehler R, Glissmeyer E et al. (2006) Genetic association of the serotonin transporter in pulmonary arterial hypertension. *Am J Respir Crit Care Med* **173**: 793–7.

Machado RD, Eickelberg O, Elliott CG et al. (2009) Genetics and genomics of pulmonary arterial hypertension. *J Am Coll Cardiol* **54**: S32–42.

Mache CJ, Gamillscheg A, Popper HH, Haworth SG (2008) Early-life pulmonary arterial hypertension with subsequent development of diffuse pulmonary arteriovenous malformations in hereditary haemorrhagic telangiectasia type 1. *Thorax* **63**: 85–6.

Massague J (1998) TGF-beta signal transduction. *Annu Rev Biochem* **67**: 753–91.

Miyazono K, Kamiya Y, Morikawa M (2010) Bone morphogenetic protein receptors and signal transduction. *J Biochem* **147**: 35–51.

Morisaki H, Nakanishi N, Kyotani S, Takashima A, Tomoike H, Morisaki T (2004) BMPR2 mutations found in Japanese patients with familial and sporadic primary pulmonary hypertension. *Hum Mutat* **23**: 632.

Morse JH, Jones AC, Barst RJ, Hodge SE, Wilhelmsen KC, Nygaard TG (1997) Mapping of familial primary pulmonary hypertension locus (PPH1) to chromosome 2q31-q32. *Circulation* **95**: 2603–6.

Nasim MT, Ghouri A, Patel B, James V, Rudarakanchana N, Morrell NW, Trembath RC (2008) Stoichiometric imbalance in the receptor complex contributes to dysfunctional BMPR-II mediated signalling in pulmonary arterial hypertension. *Hum Mol Genet* **17**: 1683–94.

Nichols WC, Koller DL, Slovis B et al. (1997) Localization of the gene for familial primary pulmonary hypertension to chromosome 2q31-32. *Nat Genet* **15**: 277–80.

Nishihara A, Watabe T, Imamura T, Miyazono K (2002) Functional heterogeneity of bone morphogenetic protein receptor-II mutants found in patients with primary pulmonary hypertension. *Mol Biol Cell* **13**: 3055–63.

Prigoda NL, Savas S, Abdalla SA et al. (2006) Hereditary haemorrhagic telangiectasia: mutation detection, test sensitivity and novel mutations. *J Med Genet* **43**: 722-8.

Remillard CV, Tigno DD, Platoshyn O et al. (2007) Function of Kv1.5 channels and genetic variations of KCNA5 in patients with idiopathic pulmonary arterial hypertension. *Am J Physiol Cell Physiol* **292**: C1837–53.

Rich S, Dantzker DR, Ayres SM et al. (1987) Primary pulmonary hypertension. A national prospective study. *Ann Intern Med* **107**: 216–23.

Roberts KE, McElroy JJ, Wong WP et al. (2004) BMPR2 mutations in pulmonary arterial hypertension with congenital heart disease. *Eur Respir J* **24**: 371–4.

Rudarakanchana N, Flanagan JA, Chen H et al. (2002) Functional analysis of bone morphogenetic protein type II receptor mutations underlying primary pulmonary hypertension. *Hum Mol Genet* **11**: 1517–25.

Runo JR, Loyd JE (2003) Primary pulmonary hypertension. *Lancet* **361**: 1533–44.

Sankelo M, Flanagan JA, Machado R et al. (2005) BMPR2 mutations have short lifetime expectancy in primary pulmonary hypertension. *Hum Mutat* **26**: 119–24.

Shi Y, Massague J (2003) Mechanisms of TGF-beta signaling from cell membrane to the nucleus. *Cell* **113**: 685–700.

Simonneau G, Robbins IM, Beghetti M et al. (2009) Updated clinical classification of pulmonary hypertension. *J Am Coll Cardiol* **54**: S43–54.

Thomson JR, Machado RD, Pauciulo MW et al. (2000) Sporadic primary pulmonary hypertension is associated with germline mutations of the gene encoding BMPR-II, a receptor member of the TGF-beta family. *J Med Genet* **37**: 741–5.

West J, Fagan K, Steudel W et al. (2004) Pulmonary hypertension in transgenic mice expressing a dominant-negative BMPRII gene in smooth muscle. *Circ Res* **94**: 1109–14.

West J, Harral J, Lane K et al. (2008) Mice expressing BMPR2R899X transgene in smooth muscle develop pulmonary vascular lesions. *Am J Physiol Lung Cell Mol Physiol* **295**: L744–55.

Willers ED, Newman JH, Loyd JE et al. (2006) Serotonin transporter polymorphisms in familial and idiopathic pulmonary arterial hypertension. *Am J Respir Crit Care Med* **173**: 798–802.

Wipff J, Kahan A, Hachulla E et al. (2007) Association between an endoglin gene polymorphism and systemic sclerosis-related pulmonary arterial hypertension. *Rheumatology (Oxford)* **46**: 622–5.

## Chapter 4

# Clinical assessment of the patient with suspected PAH and the role of cardiac catheterization

Alexander R Opotowsky and Michael J Landzberg

---

**Key points**

- The clinical evaluation of PAH includes confirmation of elevated pulmonary artery pressure as well as definition of underlying pathophysiology, aetiology, treatment options and prognosis

- An estimate of pulmonary artery systolic pressure is only one component of a complete echocardiographic assessment for PAH. Such estimates have variable accuracy and limited diagnostic and prognostic value in isolation

- Cardiac catheterization is indicated in patients with suspected PAH. Elevated mean PA pressure defines PAH, but other parameters such as cardiac output and elevated right sided filling pressures provide key prognostic information.

---

## 4.1 Introduction

Pulmonary hypertension (PH) refers to elevated pulmonary arterial blood pressure. As described in prior chapters, the underlying physiology is variable with a major distinction between PH caused by (a) elevated pulmonary venous pressure, (b) elevated pulmonary vascular (arteriolar) resistance or (c) high flow. In addition, different underlying etiologies often produce identical physiology and indistinguishable pulmonary vascular pathology. Pulmonary arterial hypertension (PAH) refers to a subgroup of PH with elevated pulmonary vascular resistance (PVR) in the absence of important pulmonary venous hypertension (McLaughlin *et al.*, 2009).

In practice, the history and physical examination along with basic testing (laboratories, electrocardiogram, and chest radiograph) often lead the clinician to obtain echocardiographic testing. An incidental finding of elevated estimated pulmonary artery pressure on echocardiography, in the absence of prior suspicion, is an increasingly frequent reason for further clinical evaluation of pulmonary vascular disease. This chapter will describe clinical findings and tests used to differentiate between the various physiologies and etiologies of PH, as well as the essential invasive hemodynamic evaluation of a patient with suspected PH.

## 4.2 The initial assessment of pulmonary hypertension

### 4.2.1 Symptoms of pulmonary hypertension

The symptoms of PAH are non-specific. Taken in conjunction with the relative rarity of PAH, this underlies the consistent delay in diagnosis. Elevated pulmonary arterial pressure itself usually does not cause symptoms. Symptoms relate to the inability to increase cardiac output (dyspnea on exertion, fatigue, pre-syncope, and syncope), elevated right atrial pressure and volume retention due to low cardiac output (edema, ascites, early satiety), or right ventricular ischemia (typical angina). Less commonly, patients may present with cyanosis or hemoptysis. Angina, pre-syncope or (especially) syncope portend poor prognosis (Peacock, 2004).

### 4.2.2 Review of other etiologies and their symptoms

History of and symptoms associated with other, frequently systemic, illnesses which predispose to or are associated with pulmonary hypertension should be elicited (McLaughlin *et al.*, 2009).

### 4.2.3 Family history

A detailed family history may provide evidence of an underlying cause of PH. As with the general history, this will be focused according to the clinical diagnosis. In addition to eliciting a history of pulmonary hypertension, information on bleeding or clotting disorders, congenital heart disease, and a pattern of sudden or premature death are important. It should be noted that a family history of premature or sudden death, often described to the family as a 'heart attack', may be due to familial PAH or another underlying diagnosis. If available, information should be confirmed with medical records and autopsy.

### 4.2.4 **Physical examination**

The examination, like the history, is useful not only to confirm findings consistent with the sequalae of pulmonary hypertension, but also to evoke signs of associated diseases.

The right ventricle sits anterior to other cardiac structures, and a palpable 'right ventricular' heave is variably present when this chamber is enlarged. Most commonly, this is best appreciated using the heel of the hand placed firmly at the inferior left lower sternal border. Right ventricular enlargement can also be palpated with the finger tips just below the xiphoid while the patient inspires deeply. In our experience, a palpable pulmonic component of the second heart sound is a specific but insensitive sign of markedly elevated pulmonary pressure.

A pulmonic opening sound is common, and the second heart sound is often widely split with normal respiratory variation. A loud P2 is more frequently present than the other markers described above. This is a subjective judgment, however, which can be confirmed when the second heart sound splits even in the apical position (after 'turning the corner'). The findings of palpation and auscultation are affected by many variables including cardiac and patient position, pulmonary parenchymal disease, thoracic deformity, and body habitus.

The pattern of jugular venous pulsations reflects the compliance of the right ventricle and may suggest tricuspid regurgitation. Palpable hepatic pulsations, likewise, support the presence of important regurgitation of the systemic atrioventricular valve.

The blood pressure response to the Valsalva manoeuvre is quite helpful in determining whether pulmonary venous pressure is elevated. In its simplest form, this only requires the clinician to describe the systolic blood pressure response to Valsalva as normal (increase lasting ≤4 beats) or sustained. The latter response argues strongly for PAOP>15 mmHg (Opotowsky et al., 2010).

Each congenital heart defect has specific findings which allow diagnosis. Other underlying disorders identified by physical findings include scleroderma (telangectasias, skin thickening), cirrhosis (jaundice, Terry nails, spider angiomata, asterixis, splenomegaly, caput medusae), neurofibromatosis (neurofibromas), intersitital lung disease (dry crackles, nail bed clubbing), and others (McGee, 2001). Airway appearance and neck circumference allow the clinician to better estimate the likelihood of obstructive sleep apnea.

### 4.2.5 **ECG**

Right atrial and ventricular hypertrophy and evidence of right ventricular 'strain' support a suspicion of long-standing elevation in pulmonary vascular resistance. As important is the presence or absence of ECG evidence for pulmonary venous hypertension (atrial fibrillation, left ventricular hypertrophy, left atrial enlargement, Q waves suggestive of myocardial infarction).

## 4.3 **Other testing**

Laboratory testing, chest radiography, lung function testing and arterial blood gas analysis are important components of the evaluation of PH, and will be discussed briefly below.

### 4.3.1 **Laboratory testing**

The first reason for laboratory testing is to determine the etiology of PH, such as connective tissue disease or HIV. Of note, a mildly elevated ANA is common with PAH and often not associated with other symptoms or signs of connective tissue disease (Thenappan et al., 2007). The second indication for lab testing is prognostic: certain serum markers such as hyponatremia or elevated BNP suggest poor prognosis with PAH. BNP provides prognostic information, but can be elevated with both right and left ventricular dysfunction so does not distinguish underlying physiology.

In the setting of a specific etiology, further laboratory testing is indicted (e.g. hypercoaguable work-up for thromboembolic PH).

Genetic testing for mutations associated with PAH is available. Discussion of this scientifically, socially, and ethically complex topic is beyond the scope of this chapter.

### 4.3.2 **Chest radiograph**

The chest radiograph provides data on gross pulmonary parenchymal disease, cardiac chamber enlargement and main and branch pulmonary artery size. The degree of distal lung vascularity (oligemic v. hyperemic) may suggest a left-to-right intracardiac shunt is present.

Restrictive lung disease can be associated with elevated pulmonary pressure. Pulmonary hypertension less commonly accompanies obstructive lung disease. The hallmark of PAH is relatively preserved lung volumes and normal flows with impaired diffusing capacity.

While obstructive sleep apnea produced generally mild PH (see below), severe obesity-hypoventilation or kyphoscoliotic lung disease can result in marked pulmonary hypertension. Significant hypercarbia will be apparent on arterial blood gas analysis. It is important to consider these entities, with a combination of history, examination, radiograph and pulmonary function testing, as part of the evaluation of PH.

### 4.3.3 **Six minute walk test**

While clinical assessment of functional status, often reported as New York Heart Association or World Health Organization functional class, is an integral part of PH evaluation, there is a great deal of variability in how clinicians make this judgement (Taichman et al., 2009). The 6 minute walk test provides more quantitative data on functional status and is an excellent method to assess changes in functional capacity (ATS, 2002). Distance walked correlates reasonably well with cardiopulmonary exercise peak $VO_2$ and is a potent inverse predictor of mortality (Miyamoto et al., 2000). It also has a role in diagnosis. For example, arterial oxygen desaturation suggests either intracardiac or intrapulmonary shunting or impaired diffusion capacity. Patients with isolated pulmonary venous hypertension rarely have frank arterial desaturation.

### 4.3.4 Echocardiography

An incidental finding on transthoracic echocardiography is one of the most common reasons for a general clinician to suspect PH as the cause of the patient's symptoms. Unfortunately, the evaluation of PH often starts and ends with PA systolic pressure estimated from the trans-tricuspid systolic velocity and pattern of IVC collapse. This is unfortunate because this parameter is neither sensitive nor specific for PAH and does not distinguish between causes of elevated pulmonary artery pressure.

PA diastolic and mean pressures can also be estimated using echocardiography (Fisher et al., 2009). The most common method to estimate diastolic pressure uses the estimated gradient between the main PA and RV outflow tract (RVOT) by measuring the trans-pulmonic valve end regurgitant velocity ($\Delta P \approx 4 \times V_2$). This value added to the estimated right atrial pressure approximates end diastolic proximal PA pressure. Mean PA pressure can be estimated using the equation in Table 4.1.

Right ventricular geometry is complex, and RV volume and function are difficult to assess with 2-dimensional echocardiography. Nevertheless, there are several simple parameters that provide relatively robust estimates of RV function in patients without congenital heart disease. Tricuspid annular plane systolic excursion (TAPSE) describes the distance traveled by the tricuspid annulus towards the probe during systole using M-Mode (or 2D) imaging. A low value (<1.8 cm) suggests right ventricular dysfunction. Other markers of predominantly right ventricular dilation or dysfunction include an RV:LV diameter ratio > 1 in the apical 4 chamber view in diastole, late systolic flattening of the interventricular septum (quantified by the eccentricity index), and an apex-forming right ventricle. There are more complex quantitative methods to estimate RV size or function such as fractional area change, but these are little used in clinical practice. The advent of 3-dimensional imaging promises improvements in echocardiographic RV quantification.

It is equally important to assess for evidence of elevated left atrial pressure or characteristics that predispose to left atrial pressure. Left atrial dilation and left ventricular hypertrophy are the most commonly measured such variables. The presence of a dilated left atrium strongly suggests long-standing left atrial hypertension. Echocardiographic estimation of left ventricular 'diastolic' dysfunction, as usually clinically implemented, is unreliable and should not be overly depended upon to determine that poor left ventricular compliance underlies a patient's elevated PA pressure. Tissue Doppler imaging may provide more specific information on left

## Table 4.1 Hemodynamic definitions and equations

**Definitions and equations:**

RA = right atrial pressure (mmHg)

MAP = mean systemic arterial pressure (mmHg)

dPAP = diastolic pulmonary artery pressure (mmHg)

sPAP = systolic pulmonary artery pressure (mmHg)

mPAP = mean pulmonary artery pressure (mmHg)

PAOP = pulmonary artery occlusion pressure (other equivalent terms: pulmonary artery wedge pressure, pulmonary capillary wedge pressure and wedge pressure)(mmHg)

BSA = body surface area ($m^2$)

HR = heart rate (beats per minute)

CO = cardiac output (l/min)

SV = stroke volume (mL/beat)=(CO × 1000)/HR

SVi = stroke volume index (mL/beat/$m^2$)=SV/BSA

WU = Wood unit (mmHg/l/min)

1 WU = 80 dyne × sec × s-5

PVR = pulmonary vascular resistance (WU or dyne × sec × s-5)

PVRi = pulmonary vascular resistance indexed to BSA (WU/$m^2$ or dyne × sec × s-5/$m^2$)

SVR = systemic vascular resistance (either WU or dyne × sec × s-5)

$cO_2$ = oxygen content of blood (mL/L)

$PaO_2$ = partial pressure of oxygen

mPAP≈0.67*dPAP+0.33*sPAP

Transpulmonary gradient (TPG) = mPAP-PAOP

$cO_2$ (mL/l) = (1.36 × [Hg] (g/dL) × $sO_2$* × 10) + ($PaO_2$ × 0.003)

$cO_2$ (mL/l)≈(1.36 × [Hg] (g/dL) × $sO_2$* × 10)

CO (Fick) = (oxygen consumption)/(arterial $cO_2$ – venous $cO_2$)

CI = cardiac index (l/min/$m^2$)=CO/BSA

CI = CO/BSA

PVR = TPG/CO

PVRi = TPG/CI

SVR = (MAP-RA)/CO

SVRi = (MAP-RA)/CI

*For the $cO_2$ calculation, the oxygen saturation is included as a decimal (e.g. 0.98). Multiplication by 10 converts units from g/dL to g/L.

atrial pressure, but lateral mitral annular velocities should be used since septal velocities are affected by right ventricular dysfunction (Ruan & Nagueh, 2007).

Finally, the RVOT pulsed-wave Doppler flow velocity envelope is an underused indicator of the state of the pulmonary vasculature. Several parameters may be evaluated. Shorter acceleration time (the time from the initiation of flow to the peak velocity) correlates with higher pulmonary artery pressure and PVR. Mid-systolic notching of the flow velocity envelope represents systolic flow deceleration in the setting of reflected pressure waves and strongly suggests elevated PVR and increased pulmonary artery stiffness (Figure 4.1).

The role of transesophageal echocardiography is limited, but is indicated for further evaluation of possible intracardiac shunt, especially for suspected sinus venosus defect.

### 4.3.5 **Other imaging**
Most patients should have high resolution computed tomography of the chest to evaluate for parenchymal lung disease, and undergo a nuclear ventilation/perfusion scan of the lungs (V/Q scan) to assess for chronic thromboembolic disease. Computed tomography pulmonary angiography is not as sensitive as V/Q scanning and is not a standard part of the initial evaluation. Magnetic resonance imaging of the pulmonary vasculature is a promising modality for evaluation of PH, but is not yet clinically widely available. In addition, MRI for evaluation of PH is not standardized, and there is wide variability between centres. In the future, MRI will undoubtedly play a larger role in diagnosis and prognostication for the array of pulmonary

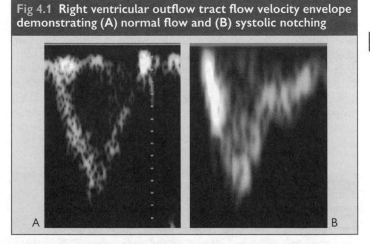

Fig 4.1 **Right ventricular outflow tract flow velocity envelope demonstrating (A) normal flow and (B) systolic notching**

hypertensive disorders. Cardiac MRI to evaluate right and left ventricular function and structure will provide further valuable data, and is an excellent modality to evaluate intracardiac or intrapulmonary shunt.

### 4.3.6 **Evaluation of sleep disordered breathing**

Obstructive sleep apnea causes intermittent alveolar hypoxia and hypercapnia, which can cause or exacerbate pulmonary vascular constriction. Other proposed etiologies for the PH associated with sleep apnea include reflex vasoconstriction with arousal and repeated Mueller manoeuvres. This may lead to mildly elevated PVR, but often the physiologic underpinning of elevated PA pressure in these patients is pulmonary venous hypertension (Hetzel et al., 2003). Patients with PH should be screened for sleep disordered breathing and, if present, should be treated appropriately. It is important to note, however, that obstructive sleep apnea does not generally cause more than mild elevations in pulmonary arterial pressure and should therefore not be assigned as the cause of moderate or severe elevations in pulmonary arterial pressure without a thorough evaluation for other causes.

## 4.4 **Invasive evaluation of suspected PH**

### 4.4.1 **When to pursue invasive evaluation**

All patients with suspected pulmonary arterial hypertension, in the absence of rare extenuating circumstances, should undergo right heart catheterization. The difficult question is, prior to invasive hemodynamic assessment who should we suspect of having PAH? Epidemiologically, the vast majority of pulmonary hypertension (i.e. elevated mean PA pressure) is associated with and due to left heart disease and consequent pulmonary venous hypertension. The non-invasive markers outlined above provide guidelines to assess the likelihood that a given patient will have pathophysiology consistent with PAH, but are no substitute for extensive experience. It should also be remembered that right heart (and, in some situations, left heart) catheterization often also provides important data to guide management in patients with other causes of pulmonary hypertension. In experienced centers, complications are uncommon and mortality is very rare (~0.055%) (Hoeper et al., 2009).

## 4.5 **Standard right heart catheterization**

### 4.5.1 **Technique**

For adults, right heart catheterization is usually performed with a single or double lumen balloon-tipped radiopaque 5–7F catheter with distance markings every 10 cm and with or without a thermistor (see below) near the catheter tip. When two fluid filled lumens are present the proximal one opens ~30 cm from the catheter tip and the distal lumen opens at the tip beyond the balloon. A third lumen is used to transmit gas or fluid from a syringe to the balloon, which usually has a capacity of 1.5 mL. This chapter will not review details of insertion of the catheter or technical details of pressure transduction or blood sampling for oximetry. Several pitfalls and suggestions are noted:

- Many pulmonary artery catheters are coated with heparin. This is an important consideration in patients with known or suspected heparin induced thrombocytopenia

- Inconsistent or unexpectedly elevated oxygen saturations should raise suspicion for intracardiac shunt

- If a 'shunt' run' is performed, samples at various levels of the circulation should be obtained in quick succession, to minimize normal temporal variation in cardiac output and, therefore, variation in venous oxygen saturations. Notably, when studied using older model oximeters, 5% of patients without an intracardiac shunt have oxygen saturation differences of up to 6% between the SVC and PA and up to 3.5% between the RA and PA (Freed et al., 2009). It is generally advisable to limit spatial variation due to streaming of blood flow (i.e. inadequate mixing) by confirming any suspected shunt with blood samples from other locations in the chambers of interest

- Hemodynamic pressure estimates should reflect the time of most neutral intrathoracic pressure, end expiration for spontaneously breathing patients. Mean pressures should not be substituted for end-expiratory pressure. In patients with labored breathing, this can overestimate true intravascular/cardiac pressures since intrathoracic pressure in such patients is not neutral at that time, and steps should be taken to limit respiratory variation. In rare cases, it may be necessary to estimate intrathoracic pressure using esophageal manometry

- It is important to confirm a true pulmonary artery 'wedge' pressure. It can be difficult to completely obstruct antegrade flow in patients with pulmonary hypertension, and even a small amount of systolic forward flow can cause inaccurately high PAOP estimates. Counter-intuitively, it is often helpful to deflate the balloon by ~0.5-1 mL, which results in forward movement of the balloon into a smaller branch vessel with a more secure seal. If necessary, small amount of air or fluid can be reintroduced to the balloon at that point, but this should be done slowly and with great caution given the small size of the occluded vessel. With care not to dissect the occluded branch vessel or to extravasate, a small amount of contrast (see discussion of wedge angiography, Section 4.8.1) may be slowly injected into the distal lumen of the PA catheter, to similarly confirm wedge position, (by demonstrating stagnant flow).

### 4.5.2 **Should a 'shunt run' be standard?**

Intracardiac shunts unrecognized prior to catheterization are a relatively uncommon cause of PH. Despite major advances in non-invasive evaluation, however, this does happen. Given the relative ease of performing oximetry at various levels of the venous circulation (usually SVC, RA, RV, PA), we perform a 'shunt run' for all PH evaluations.

### 4.5.3 **Diagnostic considerations**

There are two clinically pertinent methods to estimate cardiac output: indicator dilution and Fick techniques.

Indicator dilution involves injection of an indicator, usually cold saline, through the proximal catheter port. A thermistor, in the case of thermodilation, near the distal end of the catheter measures small temperature changes after injection of a specified volume of saline of known temperature through the proximal lumen of the pulmonary artery catheter. Using these data (quantity of indicator and area under the temperature curve), cardiac output is estimated using the Stewart-Hamilton equation. Dilution techniques are inaccurate in the setting of intracardiac shunts, and the accuracy is debated with severe tricuspid regurgitation or very low cardiac output. Measurement should be performed at least in triplicate to ensure consistent estimates. The main advantage is that dilution techniques do not require an estimate or measurement of oxygen consumption.

## 4.6 **The Fick method**

The amount of oxygen extracted from the blood is equivalent, during aerobic metabolism, to the amount of oxygen consumed by the tissues. Whatever the cardiac output, the tissues will extract a certain amount of oxygen. If the cardiac output is doubled, half as much oxygen per unit of blood will need to be extracted to support a given degree of oxygen consumption. The Fick equation uses this relationship to estimate the cardiac output using oxygen consumption (measured or assumed) and the arterio-venous difference in oxygen content.

$$\text{Cardiac output (l/min)} = \frac{\text{oxygen consumption (ml/min)}}{(\text{arterial O}_2 \text{ content-venous O}_2 \text{ content})}.$$

The blood's oxygen content is mostly composed of oxygen molecules bound to hemoglobin, with a small contribution by oxygen molecules in solution. Catheterization should be performed with the patient using their baseline supplemental oxygen, and there is a negligible absolute amount of dissolved oxygen. Therefore, the estimate of oxygen content usually ignores dissolved oxygen. Only when a patient is on very high concentrations of supplemental oxygen with very high $PaO_2$ does this have an impact on cardiac output estimates (see Table 4.1).

Oxygen consumption can be directly measured during catheterization. In clinical practice, however, assumed $O_2$ consumption is usually used. Many clinicians use a standard value of 125 mL/min/m$^2$, though empiric normative values by age, sex, body size and heart rate are available. At the extremes of body size and age, these estimates are of questionable validity even on a population scale. On an individual basis, the inaccuracy of assumed $VO_2$ constitutes one of the most important limitations of the accuracy of Fick of cardiac output estimates.

### 4.6.1 Other derived values

Pulmonary vascular resistance (PVR): this term usually refers only to the pre-venous component of resistance. Resistance describes the relationship between pressure and flow (Table 4.1), in this case between mPAP and pulmonary blood flow which approximates systemic cardiac output in the absence of intracardiac shunting.

The main hemodynamic parameters of interest in the evaluation of PH are:

(1) Mean PA pressure: this value is often calculated automatically, but can also be estimated using the systolic and diastolic pressure (Table 4.1). The presence of elevated mean PA pressure is integral to the definition of PH, but the degree of pressure elevation itself has limited diagnostic and prognostic value.

(2) PVR: elevated PVR is the primary hemodynamic feature of PAH. The hemodynamic criteria for PAH include (McLaughlin et al., 2009):
   (a) mPAP>25 mmHg
   (b) PVR>3WU
   (c) PAOP≤15 mmHg
   Notably, many patients with left-sided heart failure develop elevated PVR. After aggressive volume reduction with diuretics or hemofiltration, PAOP may improve to the normal range with sustained elevated PVR. The PVR is usually mildly elevated, but can occasionally be >4.5WU (Butler et al., 1999). While such patients are not classified as having PAH (Group I PH), elevated PVR is correlated with decreased functional ability and is an adverse prognostic sign in patients with left heart disease.

(3) Cardiac output/index: functional limitation is directly related to the systemic cardiac output and the inability to increase the

systemic cardiac output in response to demand. Systemic cardiac output is a strong inverse correlate to adverse outcomes including death in patients with PAH (McLaughlin et al., 2009).

(4) Right atrial and right ventricular end diastolic pressure: elevated RA and RVED pressure reflect right ventricular failure and are markers of poor prognosis (McLaughlin et al., 2009).

### 4.6.2 **Limitations**

While RHC is considered the clinical 'gold standard' for evaluating the hemodynamics of PH, the modality has several critical limitations. First, RHC provides only a 'snapshot' of a patient's hemodynamics at one moment in an unnatural setting. Second, symptoms tend to occur with exertion while a catheterization is performed at rest. The definition, diagnosis and management of exercise induced PH is unclear and controversial. However, there is real value in pursuing invasive hemodynamic evaluation during exercise in a subset of patients with unexplained dyspnea or other symptoms suggestive of PH or heart failure. In the absence of a formalized exercise protocol, hemodynamic manoeuvres can be useful (hand grip, leg raise, etc). Third, PVR, used clinically as a marker of overall impedance to RV output, does not provide data on the pulsatile characteristics of the pulmonary circulation. Finally, as with most tests, the quality of data and interpretation are variable and operator dependent. RHC for the evaluation of PH should be performed by experienced clinicians.

## 4.7 **Further investigations**

### 4.7.1 **Vasoreactivity testing**

It is standard practice to perform vasodilator reactivity testing in most patients with hemodynamics consistent with PAH. Acute response (see below for definition) was initially used to determine which patients would tolerate and benefit from calcium channel blockers. Vasoreactivity testing does not provide information on response to recently introduced pulmonary vasodilators. Acute response also correlates with better prognosis. With the introduction of several classes of pulmonary vasodilators, the impact of vasoreactivity on clinical management is less clear and in circumstances where calcium channel blockers are not entertained as therapy, some argue that it is no longer essential.

A variety of agents, doses and routes of administration can be used to test the acute reaction of the pulmonary vasculature to pulmonary vasodilator therapy. The most recent expert consensus document recommends use of inhaled nitric oxide (with intravenous adenosine or epoprostenol as acceptable alternatives) and defines an acute responder is a decrease in mPAP by at least 10 mmHg to

≤40 mmHg without a decline in cardiac output (McLaughlin et al., 2009). Using these definitions, very few patients are acute responders and only in a subset of this small group is this finding sustained. Of note, patients with non-familial idiopathic PAH are much more likely to be acute and long-term responders. Such response is rare among patients with other causes of PAH (e.g. congenital heart disease, sclerodema), and the utility of such testing in these patients is questionable. Vasodilator testing has the potential to cause pulmonary edema in patients with left-sided heart disease or pulmonary venoocclusive disease and should be avoided in those populations. Likewise, hemodynamically unstable patients should not undergo acute vasodilator testing, unless such testing agents are being entertained as primary therapy, both because of safety concerns during test agent discontinuation, as well as the difficulty of interpreting the findings in a state of flux.

## 4.8 Angiography

### 4.8.1 Wedge, pulmonary venous

Pulmonary wedge angiography involves hand injection of at least 2 mL of radioopaque contrast material distal to a 'wedged' pulmonary arterial catheter to opacify the distal pulmonary vasculature. The balloon is deflated, allowing contrast to flow through the pulmonary vasculature, thus outlining the pulmonary venous drainage (Figure 4.2).

Wedge angiography confirms appropriate catheter placement, and also provides a measure of the physical appearance of the branch pulmonary arteries and perfusion, the presence of pulmonary arteriovenous malformations, and possible evidence of pulmonary venous obstruction. Rapid branch pulmonary arterial tapering, longer pulmonary circulation time and decrease in background 'haze' correlate with increased PVR and more severe lung biopsy findings, at least among patients with congenital heart disease (Rabinovitch et al., 1981). As compared with CO and PVR, the angiographic appearance of the pulmonary vasculature may be more static and reflect long term pathologic changes.

### 4.8.2 Arterial

Nonselective pulmonary arterial angiography is indicated in a relatively small proportion of patients, to allow further definition of branch pulmonary artery stenosis or thromboembolic disease prior to surgical or interventional therapy. Limited subsegmental pulmonary arteriography may have greater safety, due to lower contrast load and fewer adverse effects on the RV and pulmonary arteries. For many, arterial angiography is not a routine component of the invasive evaluation of PH, as V/Q scanning (and less so, CT

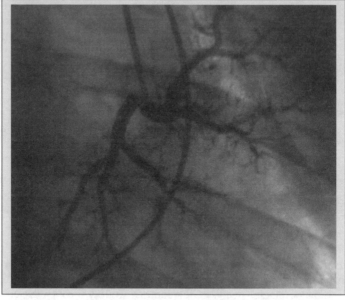

angiography) is a more sensitive test for heterogeneous pulmonary perfusion as the result of arterial or venous obstruction. However, these non-invasive techniques require spontaneous flow to distribute contrast. Catheter-based angiography can deliver contrast under guidance and pressure can be transduced at multiple sites, allowing for greater definition of location of obstruction as well for assessment of patency of vascular beds 'downstream' from the obstruction. Catheter-based pulmonary arterial and venous interventions should be limited to centers with demonstrated expertise in such procedures.

### 4.8.3 **Capillary pressure**

Pulmonary artery occlusion pressure (PAOP), often referred to as pulmonary capillary wedge pressure, is not equal to true pulmonary capillary pressure (Hellems et al., 1949). The capillaries have finite resistance and are distended by blood flow. PAOP prevents flow through the capillaries and thus underestimates capillary pressure. Capillary pressure can be estimated by inspection of the pressure transient directly following balloon occlusion of the pulmonary artery. The pressure initially decreases quickly after antegrade flow is prevented and then more slowly as capacitant blood is released from the capillaries. The intersection of these slopes (inflection) approximates true capillary pressure. These measurements are useful if pulmonary venoocclusive disease is suspected.

### 4.8.4 **Left heart catheterization**

PAOP generally correlates well with left atrial pressure in the absence of pulmonary vein stenosis or cor triatriatum. This correlation, however, depends on correct technique and interpretation of tracings. When there is uncertainty about this relationship, or when left-sided obstructive disease between the pulmonary artery and left ventricle is suspected, direct measurement of left ventricular end diastolic pressure (+/- left atrial pressure) should be obtained. Likewise, concomitant measure of RV and LV systolic and diastolic pressures with assessment of respiratory pressure variation between chambers is useful if clinical history suggests either restrictive myocardial disease or pericardial constriction.

## 4.9 **Summary**

The evaluation of suspected PH involves confirming elevated PA pressure, defining underlying physiology and etiology, providing prognostic information and determining optimal therapy. The history, physical examination and preliminary testing provide hints to the presence and cause of PH, but echocardiography and invasive hemodynamic evaluation are essential to a complete, accurate assessment of the patient with suspected PH.

# References

ATS statement: guidelines for the six-minute walk test (2002) *Am J Respir Crit Care Med* **166**: 111–7.

Butler J, Chomsky DB, Wilson JR (1999) Pulmonary hypertension and exercise intolerance in patients with heart failure. *J Am Coll Cardiol* **34**: 1802–6.

Fisher MR, Forfia PR, Chamera E et al. (2009) Accuracy of Doppler echocardiography in the hemodynamic assesstment of pulmonary hypertension. *Am J Respir Crit Cave Med* **179**: 615–21.

Freed MD, Miettinen OS, Nadas AS (1979) Oximetric detection of intracardiac left-to-right shunts. *Br Heart J* **42**: 690–4.

Hellems HK, Haynes FW, Dexter L (1949) Pulmonary capillary pressure in man. *J Appl Physiol* **2**: 24–9.

Hetzel M, Kochs M, Marx N et al. (2003) Pulmonary hemodynamics in obstructive sleep apnea: frequency and causes of pulmonary hypertension. *Lung* **181**: 157–66.

Hoeper MM, Barbera JA, Channick RN et al. (2009) Diagnosis, assessment, and treatment of non-pulmonary arterial hypertension pulmonary hypertension. *J Am Coll Cardiol* **54**: S85–96.

McGee S (2001) *Evidence-Based Physical Diagnosis*. Philadelphia: W.B. Saunders Company.

McLaughlin VV, Archer SL, Badesch DB *et al.* (2009) ACCF/AHA 2009 expert consensus document on pulmonary hypertension: a report of the American College of Cardiology Foundation Task Force on Expert Consensus Documents and the American Heart Association: developed in collaboration with the American College of Chest Physicians, American Thoracic Society, Inc., and the Pulmonary Hypertension Association. *Circulation* **119**: 2250–94.

Miyamoto S, Nagaya N, Satoh T *et al.* (2000) Clinical correlates and prognostic significance of six-minute walk test in patients with primary pulmonary hypertension. Comparison with cardiopulmonary exercise testing. *Am J Respir Crit Care Med* **161**: 487–92.

Opotowsky AR, Ojeda J, Rogers F, Arkles J, Liu T, Forfia PR (2010) Blood Pressure Response to the Valsalva Maneuver: a simple bedside test to determine the hemodynamic basis of pulmonary hypertension *J Am Coll Cardiol* In press.

Peacock AJ (2004) Clinical features. In: Peacock AJ, Rubin LJ, eds. *Pulmonary Circulation: Diseases and their treatment*. 2 ed. London: Arnold, 73–88.

Rabinovitch M, Keane JF, Fellows KE, Castaneda AR, Reid L (1981) Quantitative analysis of the pulmonary wedge angiogram in congenital heart defects. Correlation with hemodynamic data and morphometric findings in lung biopsy tissue. *Circulation* **63**: 152–64.

Ruan Q, Nagueh SF (2007) Clinical application of tissue Doppler imaging in patients with idiopathic pulmonary hypertension. *Chest* **131**: 395–401.

Taichman DB, McGoon MD, Harhay MO *et al.* (2009) Wide variation in clinicians' assessment of New York Heart Association/World Health Organization functional class in patients with pulmonary arterial hypertension. *Mayo Clin Proc* **84**: 586–92.

Thenappan T, Shah SJ, Rich S, Gomberg-Maitland M (2007) A USA-based registry for pulmonary arterial hypertension: 1982-2006. *Eur Respir J* **30**: 1103–10.

## Chapter 5

# Imaging of pulmonary arterial hypertension

Mark D Hiatt and Craig S Broberg

---

**Key points**

- Imaging provides a noninvasive means of diagnosing pulmonary arterial hypertension (PAH), determining its cause, and assessing its progression
- The pertinent imaging modalities of echocardiography (echo/ECHO), computed tomography (CT), and magnetic resonance imaging (MRI) lie along a spectrum ranging from physiologic exposition to anatomic definition
- Echo estimates pulmonary arterial (PA) pressure by measuring the velocity of flow through the tricuspid valve (TV) and is the major diagnostic tool
- CT may assist in initial evaluation of PAH by detecting pulmonary thromboembolism or intrinsic lung disease
- MR and echo are complementary, but MR excels in assessment of RV function.

---

## 5.1 Introduction

Imaging plays an important role in noninvasively diagnosing and managing PAH. The threefold goals of imaging are (a) establishing the diagnosis of PAH, (b) determining its cause, and (c) assessing its progression and estimating prognosis. In meeting these objectives, helpful modalities include echo, CT, and MRI, each with its particular strength. In general, echo excels in meeting the first goal using Doppler analysis, CT in meeting the second in structurally defining the pulmonary parenchyma and arteries, and MRI in meeting the third in elucidating right ventricular function.

Each modality provides to some extent valuable information of both form and function on a spectrum ranging from purely physiologic information on one end to anatomic detail on the other. Echo, at one end of this spectrum, delivers a wealth of physiologic data, but can be inadequate in anatomic definition, particularly of the right ventricle (RV). CT, at the other end of the spectrum, exquisitely defines anatomic structure, but conveys little about function. MR, at the spectral midpoint, yields both types of data, but not to the level of precision achievable with the other modalities.

This chapter will explore each of these techniques in turn, discussing their strengths and limitations in meeting the goals of imaging of PAH (Table 5.1). Each in its own way brings greater clarity to the evaluation of PAH, but are not all necessary in every patient. In our world of expanding imaging options but limited financial resources, the provider must justify each study by asking if a specific imaging finding can direct a clinical decision that will potentially lead to a favourable outcome for the patient.

## 5.2 Echo

### 5.2.1 Function

Echo is the mainstay of the non invasive evaluation of PAH because of its ability to estimate the PA pressure. Pressure may be estimated from the modified Bernoulli equation, $\Delta P = 4v^2$, in which $\Delta P =$ the pressure difference, and $v =$ velocity. This equation relates the velocity of blood flowing through an orifice, in this case the tricuspid valve (TV) regurgitant orifice, to the driving pressure difference across the orifice, namely between the RV and right atrium (RA) during systole.

### Table 5.1 General comparison of imaging modalities in PAH

| Modalities | Major strengths | Major limitations |
|---|---|---|
| Echo | Estimating pulmonary artery pressure, excluding left sided heart disease, portability | Accurate assessment of RV size and function, pulmonary arteries, predicting prognosis. |
| CT | Defining anatomy, technically simple, assessing lung parynchema. | Risks of radiation and contrast. Lack of physiologic data, more difficult to measure RV size and function. |
| MRI | Measuring RV size and function, excluding left sided heart disease, assessing pulmonary arteries, measuring blood flow. | Need for breath holding, longer scan times, claustrophobia, poor visualization of lung parynchema. |

Echo = echocardiography, CT = computed tomography, MRI = magnetic resonance imaging.

Thus, the peak velocity of tricuspid regurgitation (TR) can allow estimation of the pressure gradient. By adding central venous pressure (CVP), usually 5–10 mmHg estimated from visualizing the inferior vena cava (IVC), the RV systolic pressure can be quantified.

This method of estimating RV systolic pressure from TR velocity, easily measured by echo Doppler, is simple, reproducible, and reliable (Figure 5.1a, b). The accuracy of this technique has been confirmed by several studies, revealing excellent correlation with more

**Fig 5.1a Use of echo Doppler to estimate pulmonary artery pressure. The depicted TR velocities estimate pressures that are normal (top), moderately elevated (middle), and markedly elevated (bottom)**

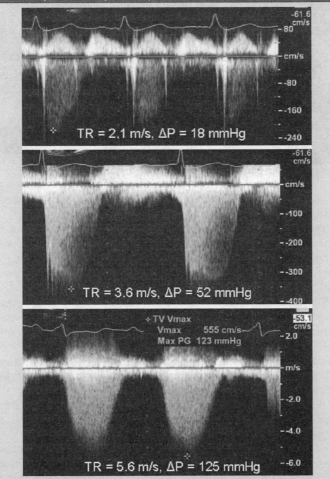

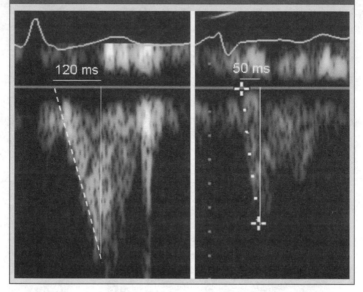

Fig 5.1b Use of echo Doppler to estimate pulmonary artery pressure. Doppler acquisition through the RV outflow tract/pulmonary artery used for quantification of acceleration time. In a normal patient (left), the measured acceleration time is 120 ms, whereas in a patient with severe PAH (right), it is 50 ms

invasive hemodynamic measurement. Some have even suggested categorizing patients based solely on TR velocity.

When an elevated TR velocity suggests PAH, alternate means of estimation may be confirmatory. First, the Doppler profile of pulmonary valvular regurgitation may estimate mean and diastolic PA pressures, with the former derived from peak early diastolic velocity and the latter from end-diastolic velocity (Table 5.2).

TR jet velocity reliably estimates pressure, but is independent of the degree of valvular regurgitation. For example, patients with marked regurgitation may have a normal TR jet velocity (<2.5 m/s), whereas others with only mild regurgitation may have an elevated velocity. The determinant of velocity is the driving pressure gradient, not the volume regressing through the valve. Likewise, the presence or absence of significant regurgitation has no bearing on PA pressure, although typically regurgitation (together with RV enlargement and dysfunction) inevitably develops as the disease progresses (Figure 5.2a).

Velocity may also be determined during exercise as an additional diagnostic criterion to help explain dyspnea on exertion in a patient with normal PA pressure at rest. Although nomograms are available,

**Table 5.2 Formulae for estimation of pulmonary arterial pressure by echo Doppler**

| Pressure estimate | Doppler derived formula |
|---|---|
| RV systolic pressure* | $4 \times (\text{TR velocity})^2 + \text{CVP}$ |
| Mean PA pressure | $4 \times (\text{peak PR velocity})^2$ |
| PA diastolic pressure | $4 \times (\text{end diastolic PR velocity})^2 + \text{CVP}$ |

\* RV systolic pressure should equal PA systolic pressure in the absence of obstruction at or near the pulmonary valve. RV = right ventricular, TR = tricuspid regurgitation, CVP = central venous pressure. PA = pulmonary artery, PR = pulmonary regurgitation.

Second, the PA acceleration time can be measured from Doppler flow into the PA (Figure 5.1b). A shorter acceleration time is indicative of possible PAH (normal >120 ms, severe PAH <60 ms).

interpretation of velocity during exercise is challenged by lack of robust criteria for a normal response in TR velocity and CVP.

The value of this modality in following established patients with worsening PAH lies not in necessarily detecting changes in pressure (due to limited accuracy at high pressures), but in defining the size and function of the RV and tracking its progressive enlargement. For this assessment, RV function from the 4-chamber view is usually subjectively interpreted (Figure 5.2a). Long axis and short axis dimensions should be measured. Objectively, measurement of the tricuspid annular plane systolic excursion (TAPSE) can be used as a guide to systolic function. Normally, the annulus is displaced over

**Fig 5.2a 4 chamber views by each modality.**
**(a) 4 chamber view by 2D echocardiography (left), and with color Doppler (right) showing severe TR**

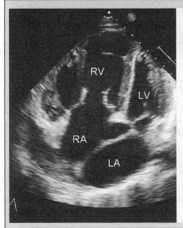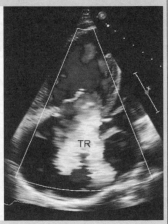

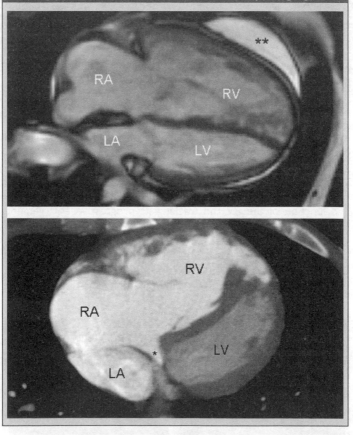

Fig 5.2b 4 chamber views by each modality.
Similar 4 chamber views from MR (upper) and CT (lower).
Note pericardial effusion on MR image (double asterisk),
dilated coronary sinus (small asterisk) and dilated right
atrium on CT. RV = right ventricle, LV = left ventricle,
RA = right atrium, LA = left atrium, TR = tricuspid regurgitation

2 cm towards the apex during systole. Doppler can also assist in
objectively assessing RV function, by way of the RV myocardial performance index (Tei index), based on Doppler-derived RV inflow
and ejection times.

When PAH is suspected by Doppler, confirmation by catheterization is mandatory. An elevated velocity without pathologic elevation
of pulmonary vascular resistance can be found in high output states
or in left-to-right shunting through an atrial septal defect. Pulmonary
vascular resistance should thus be measured invasively. Also, any
pulmonary valve stenosis (including subvalvular or supravalvular
stenosis) will raise RV systolic pressure but not PA pressure, and

thus treatable PA stenosis should not be erroneously diagnosed as PAH.

## 5.2.2 Structure

Echo also reveals structural clues in the evaluation of PAH. Structural findings to note in PAH include (a) septal deviation, (b) left ventricular (LV) size and function, (c) IVC dilatation, (d) coronary sinus enlargement, and (e) pericardial fluid. The position of the septum is dependent on the relative pressures in the RV and LV (Figure 5.3).

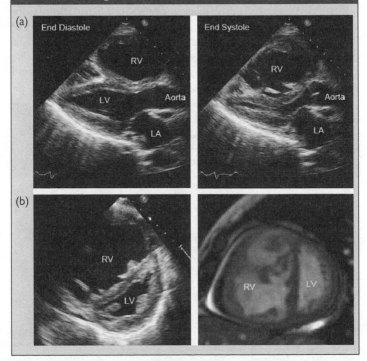

Fig 5.3 The relationship between right and left ventricles.
(a) Parasternal long axis views of a patient with PAH at end diastole (left) and end systole (right). The RV is severely enlarged. The LV is small and there is near total collapse after systole. RV = right ventricle, LV = left ventricle, LA = left atrium.
(b) Short-axis view by echo (left) and MR (right), with the latter (but not the former) depicting the RV free wall. The RV free wall is often shadowed by sternum or lung and poorly visualized by echocardiography. Note the flattened septum in both. A small pericardial effusion is also visible on this MR. RV = right ventricle, LV = left ventricle

Suprasystemic PA pressure will cause a persistent flattening of the septum throughout the cardiac cycle. In other cases, the septum is flattened during diastole, but bows towards the RV in systole when LV pressure rises higher than RV pressure. The LV may have a reduced volume from low cardiac output (CO) and septal deviation (Figure 5.3a). The presence of LV systolic or diastolic dysfunction or mitral valvular dysfunction should be excluded as causes of PAH. The IVC's diameter and pliability correlate with CVP: if the IVC is dilated over 2 cm or does not collapse (to less than typically half its caliber somewhere along its course) during normal inspiration (Figure 5.4), the CVP may be elevated to 15-20 mmHg. Positive pressure ventilation precludes this interpretation. Finally, in the setting of chronically elevated CVP, the coronary sinus may be dilated and/or a pericardial effusion may be present (Figure 5.2b).

Echo can assist with prognosis in addition to diagnosis. Many factors elucidated on echo define prognosis, including the presence of pericardial fluid, RA enlargement, and any measure of RV function. Interestingly, PA pressure estimated by Doppler is not prognostically important, as this modality is insensitive in detecting the small changes in velocity needed to track subtle deterioration over time.

### 5.2.3 Limitations

It has been demonstrated that TR jet velocity is less accurate at higher PA pressure. Thus it is an imperfect predictor of pressure and prognosis. Technical challenges preclude precise assessment of RV function, as the largely substernal RV, particularly its free wall, is difficult to image sonographically and the irregularity of this elusive chamber does not fit into simple geometric models that reliably yield

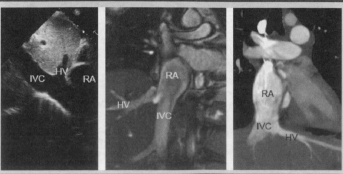

Fig 5.4 **Assessment of the inferior vena cava (IVC) dilatation by echo (left), MR (middle), and CT (right). Reflux of contrast into the IVC and hepatic veins (HV) can be seen on CT, indicative of elevated central venous pressure and/or low cardiac output. RA = right atrium**

accurate 3-dimensional volume from 2-dimensional measurements. (Figure 5.3b),

TR jet velocity usually increases with age, so cut offs of normal are not well defined. Doppler may overestimate pressure in patients with coexisting lung disease. TR jet velocity in acute pulmonary embolism (PE) must take into account the evolution of this pathology: acutely, RV dilatation and dysfunction may be present, but not necessarily pressure elevation, but over time, as the RV remodels, velocity will increase, indicating the development of PAH.

## 5.3 CT

### 5.3.1 **Structure**

At the other end of the spectrum of form vs. function CT excels in anatomic definition with unsurpassed spatial resolution, imaging the heart and lungs in exquisite detail, even depicting, for example, RV trabeculations and TV leaflets (Figure 5.2b). Yet it fails to offer rich physiologic data obtained by echo. Compared to MR, CT is less demanding in terms of operator expertise and exam time, with reconstruction of any plane possible from the raw data. The CT images should ideally be acquired with cardiac gating on a multidetector scanner using a slice thickness of 1 mm or less to give better resolution of cardiac anatomy. The patient should be able to lie flat for a few minutes and hold his or her breath for a few seconds. Contrast should be considered for enhanced visualization of the RA, RV, and main pulmonary arteries and branches, but is not necessary to make measurements or examine the pulmonary parenchyma.

Most algorithms recommend CT in the initial evaluation of PAH, mainly to exclude (a) thromboembolism and (b) intrinsic lung disease as causes. In evaluating suspected PE, CT has become increasingly accepted as the gold standard, if tailored specifically to evaluate the pulmonary arteries (requiring the timely administration of contrast). Pulmonary fibrosis, as a potential cause of secondary PAH, may also be revealed by CT (without the need for contrast). CT's exquisite anatomic detail allows such diagnoses.

In addition to evaluating for causes, CT can suggest or confirm PAH and define severity through structural assessment by revealing such cardiovascular and pulmonary abnormalities as chamber dilatation (Figure 5.2b), PA enlargement centrally and tapering peripherally, and related differential perfusion of the pulmonary parenchyma. Specifically, PAH is suggested by (a) RV and RA enlargement, (b) abnormal positioning of the interventricular and interatrial septa, (c) dilatation of the coronary sinus, hepatic veins, and IVC, with significant reflux of contrast into the latter also signifying high CVP and/or low CO (Figure 5.4), (d) dilatation of the pulmonary trunk

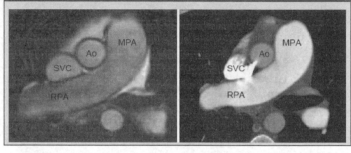

Fig 5.5 Examples of pulmonary artery enlargement as shown by MR (left) and CT (right). MR is better for evaluating distention of the pulmonary arteries (change in diameter or area through the cardiac cycle), which is reduced in pulmonary hypertension. CT is better for excluding thromboembolism in the distal segments. MPA = main pulmonary artery, RPA = right pulmonary artery, SVC = superior vena cava, Ao = aorta

(Figure 5.5) to a greater diameter than that of the ascending aorta (a caliber > 3.5 cm is highly predictive), although this criterion does not reliably predict PAH in pulmonary fibrosis, (e) peripheral arterial 'pruning,' and (f) a 'mosaic pattern' to the pulmonary parenchyma due to patchy perfusion arising from selective peripheral vasoconstriction (Figure 5.6).

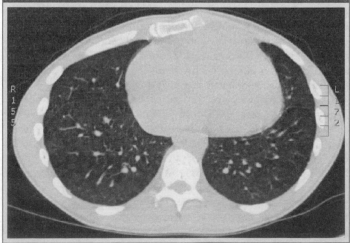

Fig 5.6 'Mosaic' pattern of lung parynchema visualized by CT, resulting from varying degrees of small artery vasoconstriction

### 5.3.2 **Function**

Physiologic data, namely RV function, can sometimes be derived from a fully gated study providing frames through the cardiac cycle. Optimal imaging on a 64-channel scanner requires a slow heart rate (best if < 65 beats per minute). Quantification of RV volume and function from only 10 frames per cardiac cycle is achievable, but with diminished reliability related to some subjective interpretation of the location of valve planes. A fully gated study also increases radiation exposure.

### 5.3.3 **Limitations**

The main limitations of CT relate to contrast and radiation. Caution is advised for patients with renal impairment or allergies to contrast, as a noncontrasted exam, reduced contrast dose, or premedication may be required. Radiation is also a concern, requiring consideration of alternate modalities, particularly in young females. For example, in diagnosing PE, ventilation/perfusion scintigraphy following normal chest radiography may be safer, delivering radiation equivalent to 800 posteroanterior chest radiographs, compared to 1,700 for CT angiography. Radiation exposure precludes routine use of serial CT for follow up evaluation.

## 5.4 **MRI**

### 5.4.1 **Function**

MRI spans the spectrum between echo in rendering physiologic data and CT in defining anatomic detail. In describing function, MRI and echo are complementary; a major strength of echo (measuring velocity) is achievable but more difficult with MRI, and one limitation of echo (measuring RV size and function) is a definite strength of MRI. Its ability to provide functional and structural assessment makes it ideal for assessing congenital heart defects, for example, in whom PAH often coexists.

MRI has become the standard for RV function analysis, and is used extensively in congenital heart disease for this express purpose. Volume is quantified by obtaining a series of short axis cine images from base to apex. From these, the ventricular area is quantified off line, and the sum of the areas multiplied by the thickness of each slice gives volume. Quantification requires some expertise and care, however, particularly in interpreting the most basal plane as it changes during the cardiac cycle. Contouring must be done conscientiously; one must distinguish atrium from ventricle near the valve planes. Some have argued for using longitudinal views where the valve planes can be more readily viewed, though the accuracy is largely unchanged. Trabeculations can be extensive in the pressure loaded ventricle such as with PAH, and different imaging laboratories debate the efficacy of including or excluding these from analysis, sacrificing reproducibility for accuracy. Serial studies in a given patient should be analyzed similarly.

Phase-contrast velocity mapping is a technique that allows determination of cardiac output and pulmonary blood flow, including differential blood flow to either lung. Shunt volume in patients with shunts can be measured. Mean PA pressure can be estimated from the pressure wave velocity, or by TR jet velocity as with echo. However, quantification of TR jet velocity can be done but not with the ease and accuracy of echo, and is not typically performed.

### 5.4.2 Structure

As with echo and CT, confirmatory findings that might be visualized with MRI include RA enlargement, pericardial effusion, and dilatation of the IVC (Figure 5.4) and/or coronary sinus, and these findings carry prognostic weight. The pulmonary arteries can also be visualized (Figure 5.5) and diameters measured. Larger diameters are expected in PAH, as with CT. MRI offers the advantage of measuring distention of the branch pulmonary arteries (area change through the cardiac cycle), and in PAH patients, the arteries appear stiffer with less distention. Large thrombi can be seen in the proximal branches, but the technique is not nearly as sensitive for small thromboemboli as CT. MR can also identify left-sided causes of PAH, such as venous occlusion and left-sided failure, or any congenital heart abnormality. Its definition of anatomy approaches that of CT for many structures but not the lung parynchema.

### 5.4.3 Limitations

Limitations of MRI relate to potential challenges with the patient's respiration, depiction of the pulmonary parenchyma and arteries, and measurement of volume. Patients must hold their breath for optimal imaging, which may be difficult for ones with orthopnea. Roughly 5% of patients will be too claustrophobic for a traditional bore scanner. MRI poorly depicts the pulmonary parenchyma and arteries (much better done by CT).

72

## 5.5 Conclusion

Echo, CT, and MRI are noninvasive means of diagnosing and managing PAH. Their particular strengths derive from their relative positions on a spectrum ranging from physiologic exposition on one end to anatomic definition on the other. Echo and CT, at opposite ends of the spectrum, yield rich physiologic information in the case of the former and exquisite anatomic detail in the case of the latter. MRI is between the two on the spectrum, and excels in quantifying RV size and systolic function. Ideally a PAH referral center will have all modalities available, and the choice of each will be determined by the unique clinical circumstances encountered with each patient.

# References

Badesch DB, Champion HC, Sanchez MA  et al (2009) Diagnosis and assessment of pulmonary arterial hypertension. *J Am Coll Cardiol.* **54**(1 Suppl): S55–66.

Bossone E, Bodini BD, Mazza A, Allegra L (2005) Pulmonary arterial hypertension: the key role of echocardiography. *Chest.* **127**(5): 1836–43.

Brecker SJ, Gibbs JS, Fox KM, Yacoub MH, Gibson DG (1994) 'Comparison of Doppler derived haemodynamic variables and simultaneous high fidelity pressure measurements in severe pulmonary hypertension.' *Br Heart J* **72**(4): 384–9.

Celermajer DS, Marwick T (2008) Echocardiographic and right heart catheterization techniques in patients with pulmonary arterial hypertension. *Int J Cardiol* **125**(3): 294–303.

Edwards PD, Bull RK, Coulden R (1998) CT measurement of main pulmonary artery diameter. *Brit J of Radiol* **71**: 1018–20.

Kim NH (2004) Diagnosis and evaluation of the patient with pulmonary hypertension. *Cardiol Clin* **22**(3): 367–73, v-vi.

Kuriyama K, Gamsu G, Stern RG, Cann CE, Herfkens RJ, Brundage BH (1984) CT-determined pulmonary artery diameters in predicting pulmonary hypertension. *Invest Radiol* **19**(1): 16–22.

Laffon E, Laurent F, Bernard V, De Boucaud L, Ducassou D, Marthan R (2001) Noninvasive assessment of pulmonary arterial hypertension by MR phase-mapping method. *J Appl Physiol* **90**(6): 2197–2202.

McQuillan BM, Picard MH, Leavitt M, Weyman AE (2001) Clinical correlates and reference intervals for pulmonary artery systolic pressure among echocardiographically normal subjects. *Circulation* **104**(23): 2797–2802.

Orrison WW, ed. (2006) *Medical Imaging Consultant.* Las Vegas, NV: OAG Publishing Co.

Torbicki A, Kurzyna M (2005) Pulmonary arterial hypertension: evaluation of the newly diagnosed patient. *Semin Respir Crit Care Med* **26**(4): 372–8.

van Wolferen SA, Marcus JT, Boonstra A et al (2007) Prognostic value of right ventricular mass, volume, and function in idiopathic pulmonary arterial hypertension. *Eur Heart J* **28**(10): 1250–7.

## Chapter 6

# Idiopathic pulmonary arterial hypertension

Stephen F Crawley and Andrew J Peacock

---

**Key points**

- IPAH is a rare but serious condition, for which there is currently no cure
- It can present at any age and is more common in females
- Left untreated survival rates are very poor
- Three classes of disease targeted therapy have recently been introduced, endothelin antagonists, phosphodiesterase inhibitors, and prostanoids
- These new treatments improve symptoms and exercise capacity, and in the case of prostanoids improve survival
- Many patients will progress to combination therapy or need surgical intervention.

---

## 6.1 Introduction

Idiopathic pulmonary arterial hypertension (IPAH) represents pulmonary arterial hypertension in its purest form. By definition, IPAH exists when an underlying cause of the PAH cannot be identified. It is a rare disease with a poor prognosis, and as discussed in Chapter 2, is characterized by luminal obliteration of small pulmonary arteries.

The overall result is increased resistance to pulmonary blood flow, rising pulmonary artery pressure (PAP), and ultimately right ventricular failure and death. In this chapter we will explore the key steps in diagnosing and managing this uncommon but serious condition.

## 6.2 **Background**

Whilst the term 'IPAH' is a relative newcomer to the medical literature, the disease it represents has been recognized for over a hundred years. In the late 19th century there were case reports of patients presenting with progressive ankle oedema, dyspnoea, and cyanosis. Post mortem examination at that time revealed obstruction of the small pulmonary arteries and right ventricular hypertrophy. However, it took a further half century for the technique of right heart catheterization to be developed, and for haemodynamic measurements to be performed in such patients. In 1951 the name 'primary pulmonary hypertension' was first used to describe cases of pulmonary hypertension without evident aetiology. The pulmonary hypertension classification has been revised several times, most recently in the 2008 Dana Point symposium, and the term 'primary pulmonary hypertension' has been abandoned and replaced with 'idiopathic pulmonary arterial hypertension (IPAH)'.

## 6.3 **Epidemiology**

Idiopathic pulmonary arterial hypertension remains a rare disease, with data from Scotland suggesting an incidence of approximately 7 per million per year. It is likely that most general practictioners and hospital clinicians will go through their entire career without seeing a new case of IPAH. However it is important to recognize that the prevalence of IPAH is increasing. In the United Kingdom pulmonary hypertension centres, the number of patients on treatment has more than doubled from 638 in 2004 to almost 1500 in 2007, i.e. 24.9 patients treated per million population. It is likely that this number will increase further as survival time increases, more patients come to medical attention and the indications for disease-targeted therapy expand.

Women are affected more commonly than men, with the female:male ratio approximately 1.7:1. Cruelly, there is a predilection for IPAH to affect otherwise normal young women of child-bearing age. The mean age for developing the condition is around 40 years, but the syndrome can occur at any age. Elderly patients often have other coexisting cardiac and respiratory disease making the diagnosis of pure IPAH more challenging.

## 6.4 **Clinical presentation**

Most patients with IPAH present with exertional dyspnoea, developing over months or years. This classical, although non-specific, symptom is thought to be due to the inability of the right heart to raise output on exertion. Chest pain, syncope, and peripheral oedema are more common in advanced IPAH, and indicate right ventricular failure. The clinical signs of IPAH, whilst subtle, can include right ventricular heave, loud pulmonary component of the second heart sound, a pansystolic murmur of tricuspid regurgitation and a right ventricular third sound. Jugular venous distension, hepatomegaly, peripheral oedema, ascites, and cold extremities indicate patients in a more advanced state with right ventricular failure at rest. Central cyanosis may also be present in advanced cases.

Unfortunately, the absence of findings on clinical examination and non-specific symptoms frequently leads to a delay in referral to the appropriate specialist centre, and subsequently a delay in diagnosis and treatment. Symptoms are often initially attributed to poor physical fitness, especially in overweight patients, and the diagnosis only becomes apparent with the development of chest pain, syncope, or oedema.

## 6.5 **Diagnosis**

To make a secure diagnosis of IPAH it is helpful to return to our definition:

- It was decided in 2008 to introduce new thresholds for mean pulmonary arterial pressure with < 21 mmHg = normal, 21–25 mmHg = borderline, and > 25 mmHg = manifest PH
- PAH also requires a pulmonary capillary wedge pressure (PCWP) ≤15 mmHg and a pulmonary vascular resistance (PVR) ≥240 dynes/s/cm5
- IPAH is PAH in the absence of any underlying cause.

As discussed in Chapter 4 the key investigation is the right heart catheter. However, other less-invasive tests can help guide the clinician towards the diagnosis of IPAH, as opposed to other forms of PAH. The ECG classically shows right axis deviation, large p-waves especially in lead II, tall R waves and ST depression in the right-sided chest leads, although this is seen in other forms of PAH. Pulmonary function tests (PFTs) often reveal normal spirometry but reduced diffusion capacity for carbon monoxide. Chest X-Ray typically shows enlarged central pulmonary arteries and right heart dilatation.

Typically the first diagnostic test to suggest the presence of IPAH is the echocardiogram. Pulmonary artery systolic pressure (PASP) is elevated in IPAH, and estimates actual pulmonary arterial pressure. Right ventricular dilatation, paradoxical septal motion, and pericardial effusion are observed in advanced cases. A CT pulmonary angiogram usually demonstrates an enlarged main pulmonary artery and reduced peripheral vascularity. The V/Q scan in IPAH may be normal, but can show heterogeneous perfusion with multiple small mismatched perfusion defects, suggesting PTE to the unaware. Six minute walk test (6MWT) at the time of diagnosis is mandatory, as baseline 6MWT values correlates with functional class, pulmonary haemodynamics, and survival.

Right heart catheterization remains the gold standard for the diagnosis of IPAH. Patients typically have a markedly elevated mean pulmonary artery pressure (PAP), usually ≥ 50 mmHg (normal <25 mmHg). A low cardiac output and high PVR indicate severe disease and poorer prognosis. If PAP is high then vasoreactivity testing in an expert centre should be done because a successful response mandates different therapy.

## 6.6 Treatment

The current therapeutic approach to PAH was introduced in Chapter 1. At present there is no cure for IPAH, so management is usually divided into general measures, disease-targeted therapy, and surgical intervention.

### 6.6.1 General measures

Oxygen therapy, anticoagulation, diuretics and management of arrhythmias have an important role in the management of IPAH (see Table 6.1)

### 6.6.2 Disease-targeted therapy

#### 6.6.2.1 Calcium channel blockers

High dose calcium channel blockers have been shown to improve survival, but only in the subset (<10%) of patients with IPAH who demonstrate a positive vasoreactivity response at right heart catheterization. Treatment is started with slowly titrated high dose calcium channel blockers (up to 900 mg/day of diltiazem or up to 240 mg/day of nifedipine). If there is no improvement after 1 month or patients are unable to achieve WHO class I or II with associated improvement in haemodynamics over 3 months, then treatment should be discontinued. Unfortunately only half of those who respond acutely will maintain a sustained response to calcium channel blockers.

#### 6.6.2.2 Endothelin antagonists

As discussed earlier, endothelin-1, a potent vasoconstrictor, has an important role in IPAH. Increased circulating levels of endothelin-1 are observed in PAH, and correlate with disease severity. Several oral agents are now available which can modify the endothelin system. Bosentan is a non-specific endothelin antagonist, blocking both the endothelin-A and endothelin-B receptors. Ambrisentan and sitaxentan are specific endothelin-A receptor blockers. Sitaxentan has now been withdrawn from the market because of a potential link with an increased risk of idiosyncratic response with life-threatening

## Table 6.1 General measures used in the management of IPAH

| | |
|---|---|
| Oxygen therapy | • Acute oxygen therapy can improve pulmonary haemodynamics in hypoxic and normoxic patients<br>• Patients with resting arterial $PaO_2$ <8kPa may be prescribed oxygen for at least 15 hrs per day<br>• Ambulatory oxygen should be offered if there is evidence of correctible desaturation of >4% to <90% on a 6MWT, with symptomatic benefit |
| Anticoagulation | • IPAH is associated with abnormalities in coagulation and fibrinolytic pathways, and impaired platelet function<br>• Anticoagulation may prevent vascular thrombotic lesions and pulmonary embolism<br>• Observational studies have suggested that wafarin therapy can improve survival in IPAH<br>• All patients should be commenced on warfarin, with target INR 2-3, unless contra-indicated |
| Diuretics | • In IPAH there is excessive afterload, resulting in right ventricular dilatation and right heart failure<br>• Diuretic therapy, often at high dosages, may benefit patients with significant fluid overload |
| Arrhythmias | • Tachyarrhythmias are poorly tolerated, and often manifest with worsening dyspnoea, syncope or right heart failure<br>• Chemical cardioversion with amiodarone is useful, although many patients will require DC cardioversion to restore sinus rhythm. If unsuccessful then ablation of accessory pathway should be considered<br>• The use of beta-blockers is contraindicated in IPAH as it limits the ability to raise cardiac output by tachycardia. |

liver toxicity. All three agents have been shown to improve exercise capacity (6MWT) and pulmonary haemodynamics when used in IPAH, whilst longer-term outcome studies have also suggested improved survival rates following bosentan treatment. The main side effect of this class of therapy is abnormal liver function. Approximately 10% of patients on bosentan will have an elevation in hepatic transaminases, although the incidence of this is lower with the other endothelin antagonists. Patients starting on this class of therapy should therefore have regular liver function tests, and increases in transaminases above 3-times normal level should result in dose reduction or even treatment withdrawal. See also Figure 6.1.

### 6.6.2.3 Phosphodiesterase-5 inhibitors
Phopshodiesterase-5 (PDE-5) inhibitors act by inhibiting the breakdown of nitric oxide's second messenger, cyclic guanosine monophosphate, thereby increasing the effect of locally produced nitric oxide.

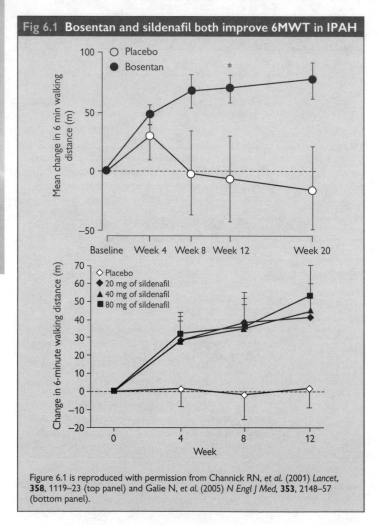

Fig 6.1 Bosentan and sildenafil both improve 6MWT in IPAH

Figure 6.1 is reproduced with permission from Channick RN, *et al.* (2001) *Lancet*, **358**, 1119–23 (top panel) and Galie N, *et al.* (2005) *N Engl J Med*, **353**, 2148–57 (bottom panel).

This results in inhibition of smooth muscle growth and pulmonary vasodilation. Sildenafil is the only PDE-5 inhibitor currently licensed for use in the UK, the recommended dose being 20 mg three times daily. If the initial response is inadequate then patients are often titrated to dosages of up to 80 mg three times daily. Treatment with sildenafil has been shown to improve symptoms, exercise capacity and haemodynamics in IPAH, whilst being associated with survival rates of up to 95% at 1 year. It is a well-tolerated agent, the main side effects being gastro-intestinal upset and postural hypotension, although concomitant use of nitrates must be avoided. See also Figure 6.1.

### 6.6.2.4 Prostanoids

Prostacyclin is a product of the arachidonic acid cascade that promotes vasodilation and inhibits vascular proliferation and platelet aggregation. Patients with IPAH have been shown to produce less endothelial-derived prostacyclin. Prostanoids are analogues of prostacyclin that are used to treat IPAH, and are now available in several forms. Epoprostenol (Flolan®) was the first approved therapy for IPAH, and remains the only treatment to have improved survival in a randomized controlled trial. An intravenous prostanoid, it requires delivery through a continuous portable infusion pump and an indwelling central venous catheter. It remains the treatment of choice for patients with advanced (Fc IV) disease, and has been shown to improve exercise capacity, patient symptoms and pulmonary haemodynamics. It has been shown to significantly improve survival in IPAH (see Figure 6.2). Prostanoid therapy is also available via the nebulized (iloprost) and subcutaneous (treprostinil—not licensed in the UK) routes. Oral prostanoid therapy is not currently approved in the United Kingdom.

Prostanoid therapy is commenced in the hospital setting, usually at low rates, e.g. 1 to 2 ng/kg/min for IV epoprostenol, titrated over several days to 5 to 10 ng/kg/min. Dose adjustment requires balancing symptom control with side effects, and will be vary with the individual. Most patients will require progressive uptitration of dosage

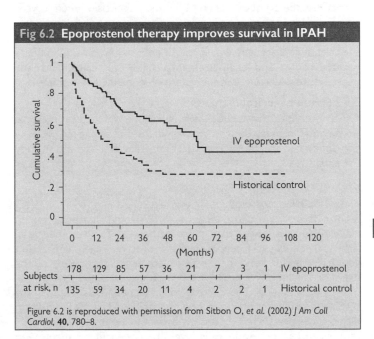

Fig 6.2 **Epoprostenol therapy improves survival in IPAH**

Figure 6.2 is reproduced with permission from Sitbon O, et al. (2002) *J Am Coll Cardiol*, **40**, 780–8.

over time. Side effects common to all prostanoids include flushing, jaw pain, diarrhoea, and body aches, and these may eventually limit the achievable dose. Serious complications related to the continuous infusion system include local catheter infections, systemic sepsis and catheter-related thrombosis. Abrupt discontinuation of intravenous prostanoid is a medical emergency as it quickly leads to severe rebound pulmonary hypertension, often fatal. Patients therefore require an intensive period of training, as they must be able to manage an infusion or frequently inhaled treatment at home.

### 6.6.2.5 *Combination therapy*

It is now common practice to use combination therapy for patients with IPAH who have deteriorated despite targeted monotherapy. The rationale is that using multiple agents will be more effective in targeting the different pathophysiolgical pathways that have been identified in IPAH. It is widely recognized that many patients will have a suboptimal response or develop tolerance to monotherapy, and it is hoped that there will be an additive or synergistic effect using combined therapy. At present the most common combination of therapy is the addition of a second oral agent, sildenafil to an endothelin receptor antagonist (ERA) or ERA to sildenafil, for patients who are WHO functional class III. For patients already on parenteral therapy it is possible to add in an oral agent, and this is indicated in the event of rapid deterioration, especially when survival time is limited. At present there is a limited amount of data on combination therapy, particularly randomized controlled trials. However the overall consensus is that it can improve symptoms, pulmonary haemodynamics, and lengthen time to clinical worsening. Currently approximately 30% of UK patients are on combination therapy.

### 6.6.2.6 *Future medical therapies*

Other potential therapeutic targets include vasoactive intestinal polypeptide, platelet-derived growth factor, the serotonin pathway and anticancer agents. Clinical trials for many of these are already underway.

### 6.6.3 **Surgical intervention**

### 6.6.3.1 *Atrial septostomy*

Studies have shown that patients with IPAH and a patent foramen ovale (PFO) live longer than those without a PFO. An inter-atrial right to left shunt can decompress the right ventricle, increase left ventricular preload and increase cardiac output, particularly during exercise. This improves systemic oxygen transport despite the arterial oxygen desaturation. The current recommended atrial septostomy technique involves trans-septal puncture followed by graded balloon dilation. The precise role of this procedure in the treatment of IPAH remains unclear, but evidence is suggestive of benefit in patients who are in WHO functional class IV with right heart failure refractory to medical therapy or with severe syncopal symptoms. It is also used in patients being considered for or awaiting transplantation.

### 6.6.3.2 Transplantation

Until the 1990s transplantation was considered the only option for some patients with IPAH in the UK. The development of disease-targeted therapy has reduced the need for transplantation, however there are still a significant number of patients who deteriorate on medical treatment, either following an initial period of clinical benefit or not. In the United Kingdom there are clear referral guidelines and set criteria for potential candidates. The potential need for transplantation should be discussed with all patients presenting in WHO functional class III, whilst patients in WHO functional class IV should be referred on presentation if they appear to be potential candidates. It is currently recommended that all patients with IPAH should have disease-targeted therapy before transplantation, and that transplantation occurs when such therapy is failing.

Single lung transplantation (SLT), bilateral lung transplantation (BLT) and combined heart-lung transplantation have all been performed for IPAH. Reduction in afterload occurs immediately after lung transplant; however improvement in right ventricular dysfunction may be significantly delayed. This can result in troublesome postoperative haemodynamic instability. Despite this complication, current practice is for patients with IPAH requiring transplant to receive BLT only. Survival after transplantation for IPAH had been reportedly among the lowest among the major lung transplant recipients. However, changes in surgical technique, perioperative care, and immunosupression have significantly improved survival. Survival rates of 86% at 1 year, 75% at 5 years and 66% at 10 years are now described in patients transplanted for IPAH.

## 6.7 Prognosis

Before the advent of disease-targeted therapy the prognosis in IPAH was dismal, with median survival only 2.8 years. This is comparable to survival in advanced breast cancer and advanced prostate cancer. Patients were frequently referred for lung transplantation at the time of diagnosis. Now patients are started on medical therapy and reassessed after several months of treatment. Follow up involves assessment of symptoms and functional class, clinical examination and evaluation of exercise capacity using 6MWT. Further investigations vary between PH centres but will usually include an assessment of RV function, using either echocardiogram, cardiac MRI, or NT-ProBNP. Right heart catheterization is not routinely repeated.

Following a period of medical therapy, poor prognosis is associated with the presence of:

- Poor exercise capacity (6MWT <380 m)
- Continued functional class III/IV symptoms
- Elevated right atrial pressure
- Low cardiac index
- Low mixed venous oxygen saturation
- Elevated NT-ProBNP
- Pericardial effusion. See also Figure 6.3.

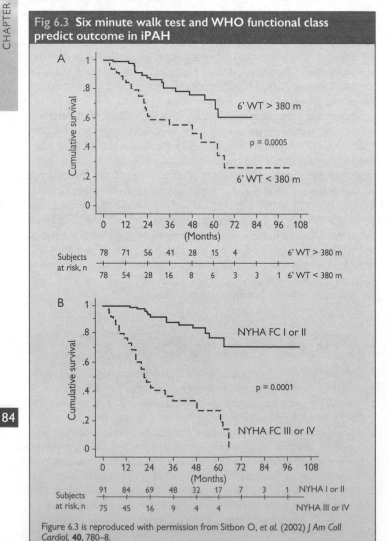

**Fig 6.3 Six minute walk test and WHO functional class predict outcome in iPAH**

Figure 6.3 is reproduced with permission from Sitbon O, et al. (2002) J Am Coll Cardiol, **40**, 780–8.

It is also worth noting that echocardiographic estimates of right ventricular systolic pressure do not predict survival, and that in advanced disease mean pulmonary artery pressure may actually fall as the right ventricle fails.

Improvements in symptoms and exercise capacity usually occur after several weeks of medical therapy, before reaching a plateau at 3–4 months. This can occur in the absence of any observable pulmonary vasodilatory response and is attributed to treatment effects on pulmonary vascular growth and remodelling. Improvement can often be maintained for several years, but there is significant variability between patients and subsequent deterioration is common. Although mortality is still high, long-term outcomes have improved within the last decade since the introduction of targeted therapies, and the 3 year survival rate has increased to 87%.

## 6.8 **Conclusion**

Idiopathic pulmonary arterial hypertension is a rare disease, but it strikes at any age, has debilitating symptoms, and shortens life expectancy. As our understanding of its pathophysiology has developed so have approaches to its diagnosis and management. Over the last 15 years we have progressed from having no specific treatment to currently having three different types of disease-targeted therapy. We have witnessed improvements in patient symptoms and exercise capacity, although survival benefits have been more difficult to achieve.

# References

Barst RJ, Rubin J, Long WA et al. and The Primary Pulmonary Hypertension Study Group (1996) A comparison of continuous intravenous epoprostenol (prostacyclin) with conventional therapy for primary pulmonary hypertension. *N Engl J Med* **334**: 296–302.

Channick RN, Simonneau G, Sitbon O et al. (2001) Effects of the endothelin-receptor antagonist bosentan in patients with pulmonary hypertension: a randomised placebo-controlled study. *Lancet* **358**: 1119–1123.

Chin KM, Rubin LJ (2008) Pulmonary arterial hypertension. *J Am Coll Cardiol* **51**: 1527–38.

D'Alonzo GE, Barst RJ, Ayres SM et al. (1991) Survival in patients with primary pulmonary hypertension. Results from a national prospective registry. *Ann Intern Med* **115**: 43–9.

Galie N, Ghofrani HA and Torbicki A et al. (2005) Sildenafil citrate therapy for pulmonary arterial hypertension. *N Engl J Med* **353**: 2148–2157.

Galiè N, Manes A, Negro L et al. (2009) A meta-analysis of randomized controlled trials in pulmonary arterial hypertension. *Eur Heart J* **30**: 394–403.

Kawut SM, Horn EM, Berekashvili KK et al. (2005) New predictors of outcome in idiopathic pulmonary arterial hypertension. *Am J Cardiol* **95**: 199–203.

McLaughlin VV, Sitbon O, Badesch DB *et al.* (2005) Survival with first-line bosentan in patients with primary pulmonary hypertension. *Eur Respir J* **25**: 244–9.

National Pulmonary Hypertension Centres of the UK and Ireland (2008) Consensus statement on the management of pulmonary hypertension in clinical practice in the UK and Ireland. *Thorax* **63**(Suppl II): ii1–ii41.

Peacock AJ, Murphy NF, McMurray JJ, Caballero L, Stewart S (2007) An epidemiological study of pulmonary arterial hypertension. *Eur Respir J* **30**(1): 104–9.

Simonneau G, Rubin LJ, Galie R *et al.* (2008) Addition of sildenafil to long-term intravenous epoprostenol therapy in patients with pulmonary arterial hypertension: a randomised trial. *Ann Intern Med* **149**: 521–30.

Sitbon O, Humbert M, Nunes H *et al.* (2002) Long-term intravenous epoprostenol infusion in primary pulmonary hypertension: prognostic factors and survival. J Am Coll Cardiol 40: 780–788.

Sitbon O, Humbert M and Jais X *et al.* (2005) Long-term response to calcium channel blockers in idiopathic pulmonary arterial hypertension. *Circulation* **111**: 3105–11.

Toyoda Y, Thacker J, Santos R *et al.* (2008) Long-term outcome of lung and heart-lung transplantation for idiopathic pulmonary arterial hypertension. *Annals Thorac Surg* **86**: 1116–22.

Van Wolferen SA, Grunberg K, Vonk Noordegraaf A (2007) Diagnosis and management of pulmonary hypertension over the past 100 years. *Resp Med* **101**: 389–98.

## Chapter 7

# Chronic thromboembolic pulmonary hypertension (CTEPH)

David P Jenkins, Nicholas W Morrell, Karen Sheares and Joanna Pepke-Zaba

## Key points

- CTEPH is one of the most prevalent forms of pulmonary hypertension (PH) and should be considered in all cases with unexplained PH
- Patients with persistent breathlessness following pulmonary emboli should be further investigated and referred to an experienced PH centre
- Patients with CTEPH should receive lifelong anticoagulation and be considered for the treatment with pulmonary endarterectomy (PEA)
- Pulmonary endarterectomy is the treatment of choice in selected cases and may be curative with normalization of pulmonary artery pressures and significant symptomatic and prognostic benefit
- In selected CTEPH patients not suitable for surgery or patients with residual PH after PEA, treatment with pulmonary hypertension targeted drug therapy may be considered by experienced PH centres.

## 7.1 Introduction

Chronic thromboembolic pulmonary hypertension (CTEPH) results from obstruction of the pulmonary vascular bed by non-resolving thromboemboli. These may completely occlude the lumen or form different grades of stenosis, webs and bands. Interestingly, in the non-occluded areas, a pulmonary arteriopathy indistinguishable from that of pulmonary arterial hypertension can develop. CTEPH can be found in patients without any previous clinical episode of acute pulmonary embolism or deep venous thrombosis. CTEPH is defined as pre-capillary pulmonary hypertension (mPAP >25 mmHg, pulmonary capillary wedge pressure <15 mmHg, PVR >2 Wood Units) with persistent perfusion defects. In the absence of treatment, CTEPH has historically had a poor prognosis, although in the majority of cases, it can now be treated effectively with PEA surgery.

## 7.2 Epidemiology

The prevalence and incidence of CTEPH are difficult to ascertain. Recent follow-up studies in patients presenting with acute pulmonary embolism (PE) give an estimates of cumulative incidence ranging from 0.8% to 3.8%. Given that acute venous thromboembolism (VTE) is as common as 1/1000 population per year, the annual incidence of CTEPH following VTE may be of the order of 8–40 cases/ million population. Moreover, given that CTEPH may present some time following an acute event and also about 60% of patients with CTEPH have not had a documented VTE, the results from these relatively short studies are likely to represent an underestimate. In a study of 469 patients diagnosed prospectively with CTEPH in UK PH Centres between 2001 and 2005, the calculated incidence in 2005 was 1.75 cases/year/million. This is a conservative estimation as it excluded patients who had been diagnosed but not referred to a PH centre.

## 7.3 Pathogenesis of CTEPH

CTEPH can be considered as a failure of resolution of the clot burden following acute PE. Treatment of patients with anticoagulation effectively prevents the generation of further thrombus. Fibrinolysis of clot is then achieved by endogenous pathways. In the initial 'early' phase, thrombus resolution probably results from a combination of thrombus fragmentation and endogenous fibrinolysis. In the majority of patients this leads to complete clot resolution. However, a significant proportion of patients have continuing clot beyond this early phase. Further resolution beyond this point is likely to rely on a process of clot organization and neovascularization, during which the obstructed vessel becomes recanalized and vessel patency is restored.

### 7.3.1 Abnormalities of coagulation and fibrinolysis

Most studies have failed to show any significant association between hereditary thrombophilia and CTEPH, despite the prevalence of these in deep vein thrombosis (DVT) and VTE. Elevated Factor VIII levels have also been demonstrated in CTEPH, compared with controls. Furthermore, levels failed to normalize following successful PEA surgery. The persistent elevation of Factor VIII following PEA surgery suggests that elevated Factor VIII levels may play a causal role in the development of CTEPH and are not simply a non-specific secondary response to abnormal pulmonary artery pressures.

During platelet activation, Factor V is released from platelet granules and is subsequently cleaved by thrombin to form activated Factor Va. This in turn acts as a co-factor with Factor Xa in the production of thrombin from prothrombin. Although a number of genetic variants of Factor V exist, the most clinically relevant is Factor V Leiden. Many studies have demonstrated that possession of the Factor V Leiden allele is strongly associated with an increased risk of VTE. However, limited studies of CTEPH subjects, suggest that the mutation is not such a prominent feature in this disease.

Both quantitative and qualitative defects in protein C and S activity have been described, and have been reported to increase the risk of VTE. However, only one study has examined the prevalence of these defects in CTEPH. This study demonstrated a slightly higher, but non-significant, prevalence of protein C deficiency and no higher prevalence of protein S deficiency in patients with the condition.

Antiphospholipid antibodies (aPL) are present in a number of conditions where they represent autoantibodies directed against cell membrane constituents. In high titres, their occurrence is associated with an increased risk of both arterial and venous thromboses. A number of studies have reported an association between aPLs and CTEPH, with prevalence varying between 10% and 20%.

Fibrinogen plays a pivotal role in balancing haemostasis, by acting as a substrate for both the coagulation and fibrinolytic systems. Abnormalities affecting fibrinogen levels but also fibrinogen function have been described. Clearly, prothrombotic abnormalities of fibrinogen are of interest in CTEPH, as this offers one potential mechanism by which thrombus may persist following an acute embolic event. A recent in vitro study highlighted this possibility by demonstrating that fibrin derived from patients with CTEPH was more resistant to lysis compared to controls. An association between polymorphism of the fibrinogen Aα (Thr312Ala) chain and CTEPH has been reported recently. The same polymorphism is more closely associated with PE, rather than DVT perhaps indicating that this polymorphism alters the structure of fibrin and predisposes clot to fragmentation and embolism.

### 7.3.2 Secondary arteriopathy

CTEPH patients often display severe pulmonary hypertension that cannot be fully explained purely by the degree of pulmonary vascular obstruction visible on conventional imaging. In these cases the increased pulmonary vascular resistance may be due to distal obstructive thrombotic lesions situated beyond the subsegmental level, but also due to arteriopathic changes at a pre-capillary level. These distal changes are responsible for the proportion of patients who have persisting pulmonary hypertension following PEA and may be amenable to targeted PAH drug therapy.

### 7.3.3 Risk factors and associated medical conditions

A history of VTE, splenectomy, thrombophilia, anti-phospholipid antibodies, ventriculo-atrial shunt, chronic central intravenous lines, inflammatory bowel disease, osteomyelitis, malignancy, thyroid replacement therapy, increase the likelihood of CTEPH. The mechanisms linking these conditions to CTEPH have not been fully explored, but chronic inflammation or chronic bloodstream infection may play a critical role.

## 7.4 Diagnostic assessments in CTEPH: making a diagnosis and determining suitability for surgery

The diagnosis of CTEPH should be considered in a patient with unexplained pulmonary hypertension or persistent breathlessness after VTE and lead to definitive investigations as shown in Figure 7.1.

Once a diagnosis of CTEPH is made, determining whether a patient is a candidate for PEA involves additional investigations and careful assessment by an experienced multidisciplinary team including PEA surgeons.

The physical examination in a patient with CTEPH is similar to that of any patient with PH, except for pulmonary flow murmurs. These are soft 'bruits' heard over the lung fields in areas corresponding to partially occluded pulmonary arteries.

Routine haematological and biochemical tests are usually unremarkable. Pulmonary function tests are generally within the normal range or show only a mild restrictive pattern resulting from parenchymal scarring. The diffusing capacity for carbon monoxide may be normal or reduced.

Echocardiography may be useful for the follow up of survivors of acute pulmonary embolism who showed signs of pulmonary hypertension or right ventricular dysfunction.

Chest radiography may reveal focal areas of hypovascularity or wedge-shaped peripheral infiltrates consistent with pulmonary infarcts, but is often unremarkable.

Persistent segmental perfusion defects with normal or near normal ventilation on V/Q scan confirms the diagnosis. The multislice CT and MRA imaging are widely used (Figure 7.2), but pulmonary

## Fig 7.1 Diagnostic work-up for CTEPH

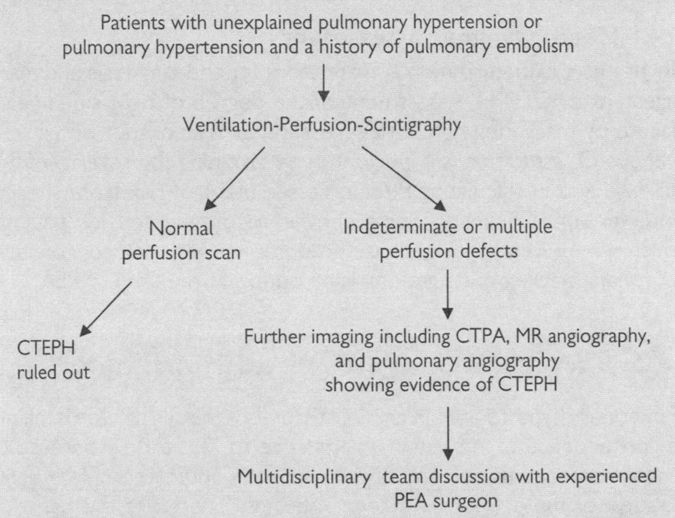

Patients with unexplained pulmonary hypertension or
pulmonary hypertension and a history of pulmonary embolism

↓

Ventilation-Perfusion-Scintigraphy

Normal
perfusion scan

Indeterminate or multiple
perfusion defects

↓

CTEPH
ruled out

Further imaging including CTPA, MR angiography,
and pulmonary angiography
showing evidence of CTEPH

↓

Multidisciplinary team discussion with experienced
PEA surgeon

Reproduced with permission from Hoeper, Barberà, Channick, *et al.* Diagnosis, assessment,
and treatment of non-pulmonary arterial hypertension pulmonary hypertension. *Journal of
the American College of Cardiology,* **51**, 1. Copyright Elsevier © 2009.

## Fig 7.2 CT of patient with thrombo-embolic PAH

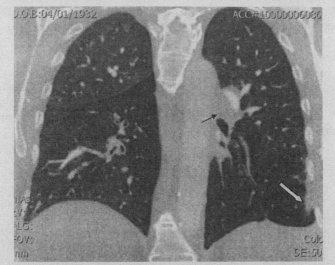

A coronal reconstruction from a CT pulmonary angiogram shows:
1. Mosaic attenuation pattern of the lung parenchyma typical of occlusive vascular disease.
2. A large thrombus (*black arrow*) almost filling the lumen of the left pulmonary artery.
3. A peripheral area of scarring (*white arrow*) in the left lower lobe and blunting of the left
costo-phrenic angle—the sequelae of previous pulmonary infraction.

angiography is still considered the 'gold standard' diagnostic tool in the work-up of CTEPH (see Chapter 5).

### 7.4.1 Haemodynamic assessment

Right heart catheterization is mandatory for the diagnosis and management of CTEPH. Assessment of the degree of right-sided heart failure by measuring right atrial pressure, cardiac output, and mixed venous $O_2$ saturation is important in determining the severity of the disease and in calculating PVR for assessment of risk from surgical intervention. Coronary angiography is recommended for patients over 40–45 years being considered for surgery, as concomitant coronary artery bypass grafting is an option at the time of PEA.

## 7.5 Surgical management and outcomes

Pulmonary hypertension in chronic thromboembolic disease is mainly a consequence of intraluminal resistance to blood flow because of thrombus organization and fibrous stenosis and/or complete obliteration of the pulmonary artery branches. Therefore the basis for the operation is a mechanical removal of the physical obstruction by an endarterectomy within the superficial media of the arterial wall. This is different from the simple 'embolectomy' performed for acute pulmonary embolus.

### 7.5.1 Types of disease

Although pre-operative imaging is very important in deciding who will benefit from endarterectomy, the ease of dissection and true extent of clearable disease can only determined at operation. The disease has been classified into four subgroups based on the operative findings: patients with types 1 and 2 disease (central lobar and segmental obstruction) deriving more benefit from endarterectomy at lower peri-operative risk, than those with more distal segmental disease (type 3) or those misdiagnosed who have idiopathic disease rather than CTEPH (type 4).

### 7.5.2 Pulmonary vascular resistance

Overall, the key determinant of operability is the correlation between the degree of visible disease in imaging studies and PVR. The absolute pre-operative and resultant post-operative PVR are the main factors that determine outcome after endarterectomy. Mortality following endarterectomy may be five to ten fold higher in patients with a pre-operative PVR > 1200 dyne/s/cm$^{-5}$. A post-operative residual PVR of > 500 dyne/s/cm$^{-5}$ is a risk factor for in-hospital mortality.

### 7.5.3 Surgical technique

The fundamental aim of the surgery is to perform a full endarterectomy bilaterally. The operation is performed via a median sternotomy with cardiopulmonary bypass (CPB), cooling to 20°C, and right and left pulmonary arteriotomies within the pericardium. Adequate visualization for distal dissection necessitates reduction in bronchial arterial collateral return to the pulmonary arteries. Traditionally this has been achieved by periods of complete deep hypothermic circulatory arrest (DHCA) for up to 20 minutes per side and this technique remains the standard teaching. The endarterectomy plane is raised using a scalpel and spatula and dissection proceeds within the superficial media of the vessel wall that is only 1–2 mm in thickness. By the use of a sucker-dissector, the plane can be extended circumferentially and then distally by careful traction as far as possible with the intention of tracing the endarterectomy into all the affected segmental or subsegmental vessels. A cast of the inner layer of the pulmonary arterial tree is then dissected free moving towards the periphery (Figure 7.3).

After completion of the endarterectomies, the patient is rewarmed slowly on full CPB. Any concomitant cardiothoracic surgical procedures can be completed during this phase of the operation. The patient is then weaned from CPB keeping right sided filling pressures low, guided by invasive haemodynamic monitoring.

### 7.5.4 Post-operative care and haemodynamic changes

There is early post operative haemodynamic improvement with an immediate fall in mean PA pressure by approximately 50%, and reduction in PVR to approximately one third of the preoperative

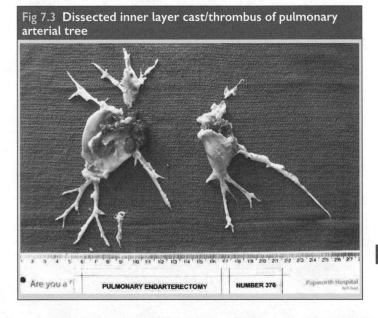

Fig 7.3 **Dissected inner layer cast/thrombus of pulmonary arterial tree**

PULMONARY ENDARTERECTOMY    NUMBER 376    Papworth Hospital

level in majority of patients. Many patients can be extubated by the first post operative day. Most of the general principles of postoperative cardiac surgical care apply and in addition it is important to avoid any factors that may increase PVR. An aggressive diuresis is maintained in the first 24 to 48 hours post-op. In the absence of post-operative bleeding, anticoagulation is usually commenced within the first two days.

### 7.5.5 Mortality and complications

Many units have reported excellent early results after pulmonary endarterectomy with an overall in-hospital mortality of 5% or less in most experienced centres. The two most serious complications following pulmonary endarterectomy are residual pulmonary hypertension and reperfusion lung injury. The latter is a form of acute lung injury, and is present to some extent in up to 15% of patients. Patients with severe reperfusion injury may benefit from veno-veno ECMO support and the sickest patients with significant residual PH may benefit from central veno-arterial ECMO in the first few days following surgery.

### 7.5.6 Long-term follow up and survival after PEA

Less data is available on longer term follow up. In the UK we review all patients at three months and one year after endarterectomy. In a recent review of 230 patients we demonstrated a significant increase in six-minute walk distance from 276.3 ± 17 to 394.7 ± 15 m by one year. NYHA class also improves significantly after surgery (see Figure 7.4). Long term survival is also significantly improved from that expected from historical cohorts (see Figure 7.5). Pulmonary endarterectomy may be curative in a large number of patients.

## 7.6 Medical therapy

### 7.6.1 Anticoagulation

CTEPH patients should receive lifelong anticoagulation adjusted to a target international ratio between 2.0 and 3.0. When the disease

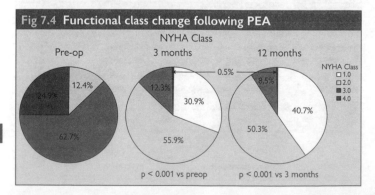

Fig 7.4 Functional class change following PEA

NYHA Class

Pre-op — 3 months — 12 months

NYHA Class
□ 1.0
□ 2.0
■ 3.0
■ 4.0

Pre-op: 12.4%, 24.9%, 62.7%

3 months: 0.5%, 12.3%, 30.9%, 55.9%

12 months: 8.5%, 40.7%, 50.3%

p < 0.001 vs preop      p < 0.001 vs 3 months

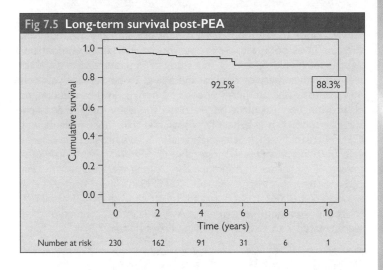

**Fig 7.5** Long-term survival post-PEA

92.5%

88.3%

Number at risk   230   162   91   31   6   1

is fully established, significant regression of pulmonary hypertension from anticoagulation is not expected.

### 7.6.2 When is medical therapy for CTEPH appropriate?

There is no licensed medical therapy for CTEPH. As the histopathological changes typical of PAH are seen in patients with CTEPH, the PAH disease-modifying therapies might be considered in selected patients. Data from clinical trials in CTEPH are limited. There is one multicentre randomized clinical trial, BENEFiT, which showed improvement in PVR, CI, and brain natriuretic peptide, but no change in exercise capacity after 16 weeks treatment with bosentan and one small single-centre RCT showing similar results with sildenafil. The majority of reports are from small uncontrolled studies with prostanoids, endothelin receptor antagonists, and phosphodiesterase-5 inhibitors. Specific PAH drug therapy may play a role in selected CTEPH patients, mainly for three different scenarios: 1) if patients are not considered candidates for surgery (elevation of PVR out of proportion to what is attributable to mechanical thrombus obstruction signals significant levels of arteriopathy); 2) if pre-operative treatment is deemed appropriate to improve haemodynamics; and 3) if patients present with symptomatic residual/recurrent PH after pulmonary endarterectomy surgery. In open-label studies, there was statistically significant improvement in functional status as measured with 6 min walking test (6MWT) after 1 year of treatment with disease-modifying therapies. There is a further need for prospective RCTs to clarify the role of targeted therapies in the treatment of CTEPH. In appropriate patients, lung transplantation may be considered.

### 7.6.3 **Survival**

Survival prior to the modern treatment era with disease-modifying therapies was poor with 3-year survival as low as 10% in patients with an mPAP of >30 mmHg. In a study of 35 patients who were not treated with surgery or medical therapies, 2-year survival was only 10% in those with an mPAP of over 50 mmHg. In these studies, no clear distinction was made between the survival in surgical and non-surgical cohorts. It is generally recognized that most patients with CTEPH treated with anticoagulation alone have progressive disease.

Survival in patients with inoperable CTEPH or persistent PH following PEA appears to be improving. A long-term follow-up study of a national cohort of patients with CTEPH in UK PH centres in the period 2003–2006, showed 1- and 3-year survival of 83% and 76%, for those with inoperable disease. A significant percentage of them were treated with disease-modifying drugs (Figure 7.6).

## 7.7 **Conclusions**

CTEPH is one of the most prevalent forms of PH. Thrombotic lesions in the pulmonary vasculature and subsequent failures of resolution probably initiate the disease. The disease could be described as two compartmental: obstruction of proximal vasculature and a small vessel component with histological presentation similar to pulmonary arterial hypertension. While PEA is the treatment of choice for CTEPH, evidence is accumulating for the potential use of medical therapies for those who are not suitable for surgery. It is important

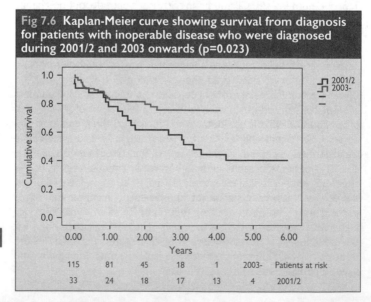

Fig 7.6 **Kaplan-Meier curve showing survival from diagnosis for patients with inoperable disease who were diagnosed during 2001/2 and 2003 onwards (p=0.023)**

to identify patients with this treatable condition because outcome has improved dramatically in the modern treatment era.

# References

Condliffe R, Kiely DG, Gibbs JS et al. (2008) Improved outcomes in medically and surgically treated chronic thromboembolic pulmonary hypertension. *Am J Respir Crit Care Med* **177**: 1122–7.

Dartevelle P, Fadel E, Mussot S et al. (2004) Chronic thromboembolic pulmonary hypertension. *Eur Respir J* **23**: 637–48.

Freed D, Thomson B, Tsui S et al. (2008) Functional and haemodynamic outcome 1 year after pulmonary thromboendarterectomy. *Eu J Cardiothoracic Surg* **34**: 525–30.

Hoeper M, Barbera J, Channick R et al. (2009) Diagnosis, assessment, and treatment of non-pulmonary arterial hypertension pulmonary hypertension. *J Am Coll Cardiol* **54**: S85–96.

Jais X, Ioos V, Jardim C et al. (2005) Splenectomy and chronic thromboembolic pulmonary hypertension. *Thorax* **60**: 1031–4.

Jais X, D'Armini AM, Jansa P et al. (2008) Bosentan for treatment of inoperable chronic thromboembolic pulmonary hypertension: BENEFiT (Bosentan Effects in iNopErable Forms of chronIc Thromboembolic pulmonary hypertension), a randomized, placebo-controlled trial. *J Am Coll Cardiol* **52**: 2127–34.

Jamieson SW, Kapelanski DP, Sakakibara N et al. (2003) Pulmonary endarterectomy: experience and lessons learned in 1,500 cases. *Ann Thorac Surg* **76**: 1457–62.

Morris T, Marsh J, Chiles P et al. (2009) High prevalence of dysfibrinogenaemia among patients with chronic thromboembolic pulmonary hypertension. *Blood* **114**: 1929–36.

Pengo V, Lensing A, Prins M et al. (2004) Incidence of chronic thromboembolic pulmonary hypertension after pulmonary embolism. *New Engl J Med* **350**: 2257–64.

Riedel M, Stanek V, Widimisky J et al. (1982) Long-term follow-up of patients with pulmonary thromboembolism: late prognosis and evolution of hemodynamic and respiratory data. *Chest* **81**: 151–8.

Suntharalingam J, Machado RD, Sharples LD et al. (2007) Demographic features, BMPR2 status and outcomes in distal chronic thromboembolic pulmonary hypertension. *Thorax* **62**: 617–22.

Suntharalingam J, Goldsmith K, van Marion V et al. (2008) Fibrinogen Aalpha Thr312Ala polymorphism is associated with chronic thromboembolic pulmonary hypertension. *Eur Respir J* **31**: 736–41.

Suntharalingam J, Treacy CM, Doughty NJ et al. (2008) Long term use of sildenafil in inoperable chronic thromboembolic pulmonary hypertension. *Chest* **134**: 229–36.

Thistlethwaite PA, Mo M, Madani MM et al. (2002) Operative classification of thromboembolic disease determines outcome after pulmonary endarterectomy. *J Thorac Cardiovasc Surg* 124: 1203–11.

Wagenvoort CA (1995) Pathology of pulmonary thromboembolism. *Chest* **107**: 10S–7S.

## Chapter 8

# Connective tissue disease associated pulmonary arterial hypertension

Benji E Schreiber, Christopher J Valerio and
J Gerry Coghlan

## 8.1 Introduction

Connective tissue diseases (CTD) are a diverse group of multisystem disorders linked by common clinical and pathological features. Although uncommon, the mortality associated with these autoimmune conditions is substantial due to the relatively high frequency of organ based complications, including pulmonary arterial hypertension (PAH). In randomized therapeutic trials of PAH, the second largest subpopulation has been patients with connective tissue disease associated pulmonary arterial hypertension (CTDPAH) (Rubin et al., 2002, Simmoneau et al., 2002, Olschewski et al., 2002, Galie et al., 2002, Barst et al., 2004, Ghofrani et al., 2004).The reason for this is that CTDPAH is relatively common in the context of this rare condition, and screening programmes are relatively well advanced in many countries. The pulmonary hypertension specialist needs a good working knowledge of the connective tissue diseases associated with pulmonary hypertension as the prognosis and management of these patients is, in important respects, different to that of idiopathic pulmonary hypertension.

## 8.2 Epidemiology

Considerable controversy continues to exist about the prevalence and incidence of PAH in various forms of CTD. Data from the post marketing surveillance survey on bosentan and the UK national survey confirm that though CTD as a whole represents the second largest subgroup of patients with PAH, this is almost exclusively driven by the SSc population (Humbert, 2005, Condliffe et al., 2009). Estimates of the prevalence of systemic sclerosis (SSc) associated PAH vary from 2.6% to 60% (Battle et al., 1996, Yoshida et al., 2001), but national studies have shown that the reality is, allowing for the limitations of screening tools, less than 10% (Hachulla *et al.*, 2005). Similarly, in rheumatoid arthritis (RA) where clinical experience shows that PAH is rare the published estimate had suggested that the prevalence may be 20% (Dawson *et al.*, 2000), but again the UK national survey has shown that in fact RA is very rarely associated with PAH (Condliffe *et al.*, 2009). Systemic lupus erythematosus (SLE) is a further important subgroup, although less than 1% of individuals with SLE develop PAH (Humbert, 2005). The second largest group is mixed connective tissue disease, where due to a lack of standardized definitions the total population is unclear, so the frequency of this complication is unknown. The development of PAH in the absence of significant interstitial lung disease has been reported in primary Sjögren's syndrome, dermatomyositis and polymyositis but the association is too infrequent for an accurate estimation of PAH prevalence in these conditions (Launay *et al.*, 2007, Minai, 2009).

Given the inherent limitations of currently available screening techniques, the only CTDs in which the prevalence justifies routine screening are systemic sclerosis and mixed connective tissue disease (Galie *et al.*, 2009a, McLaughlin *et al.*, 2009), though the recommendations in this regard have been downgraded as a result of the low yield observed in the ItinérAIR cohort follow-up project (Hachulla *et al.*, 2009a). For reference purposes epidemiological studies of PAH in SSc, SLE and mixed connective tissue disease (MCTD) are listed in Tables 8.1–8.3.

An important limitation of all these estimates is the reliance on echocardiographic screening to determine which patients should proceed to catheterization. It is clear that patients with significant pulmonary hypertension may have completely reassuring echocardiography (Mukerjee *et al.*, 2004)). The DETECT study is a cross-sectional and longitudinal study of patients with scleroderma spectrum diseases, by catheterization (Siebold *et al.*, 2008). This is a multinational study recruiting patients believed to be at high risk of SSc associated pulmonary hypertension (>3 years from diagnosis with gas transfer < 60% of predicted). 500 patients will be recruited, all will undergo a battery of screening tests and then cardiac catheterization. Those in whom pulmonary hypertension is not diagnosed will be followed up with repeat screening annually and catheterization after 3 years. Once completed this will provide prospective evidence on the proportion of the scleroderma population that have pulmonary hypertension, despite normal echocardiography. A true estimate of the prevalence of PAH and other forms of pulmonary hypertension will then be possible. Patients without pulmonary hypertension at study entry will undergo repeat catheterization at 3 years, allowing for the first time a true understanding of the incidence of PAH in SSc patients and thus calculations of the accuracy and cost-efficacy of possible screening programmes.

Table 8.1 **Systemic sclerosis**

| First author | Year | Population size | Diagnostic criteria | Prevalence |
|---|---|---|---|---|
| Battle | 1996 | 17 | Cardiac catheter (PVR based) | 65% |
| Vlachoyiannopoulos | 2000 | 203 | Cardiac catheter or echo | 2.5% |
| Yoshida | 2001 | 3778 | Cardiac catheter or echo | 2.6% |
| Mukerjee | 2003 | 722 | Cardiac catheter | 12% |
| Wigley | 2004 | 586 (prospective cohort) | eRVSP >40mmHg eRVSP >30mmHg | 13% 42% |
| Hachulla | 2004 | 617 | Cardiac catheter | 7% |
| Marasini | 2005 | 51 | ePASP >35mmHg | 20% |
| Hunzelmann | 2008 | 1158 | Cardiac catheter or eRVSP >40mmHg | 7% |

Table 8.2 **Systemic lupus erythematosis**

| Author | Year | Population size | Diagnostic criteria | Prevalence |
|---|---|---|---|---|
| Winslow | 1995 | 28 | ePASP >30mmHg | 43% |
| Li | 1999 | 419 | ePASP >30mmHg | 4% |
| Pan | 2000 | 786 | ePASP | 4.3% |
| Yoshida | 2001 | 9015 | Echo or catheter findings | 0.9% |
| Tanaka | 2002 | 194 | ePASP | 6% |
| Marasini | 2005 | 33 | ePASP >35mmHg | 6.1% |
| Prabu | 2009 | 288 | ePASP >30mmHg | 4.2% |

Table 8.3 **Mixed connective tissue disease**

| Author | Year | Population size | Diagnostic criteria | Prevalence |
|---|---|---|---|---|
| Alpert | 1983 | 17 | Catheter (PVR only) | 64% |
| Michels | 1997 | 224 | Various | 1% |
| Yoshida | 2001 | 1651 | Echo or catheter | 5% |
| Wigley | 2004 | 89 (prospective cohort) | ePASP >40mmHg | 7% |
| Marasini | 2005 | 4 | ePASP >35mmHg | 75% |
| Hunzelmann | 2008 | 162 includes Sjögren's overlap | Cardiac catheter/eRVSP >40mmHg | 8% |

## 8.3 Overview of the diagnosis and clinical features of connective tissue diseases

Physicians managing patients with pulmonary hypertension need to be able to identify the underlying conditions leading to pulmonary hypertension. CTD influences not just prognosis, but determines treatment choice and introduces complexities into the investigation and management of clinical worsening events. A breakdown of the relative prevalence of the CTDs seen in association with PAH is shown in Figure 8.1 (Condliffe, 2009).

### 8.3.1 Systemic sclerosis (scleroderma)

Systemic sclerosis is a multisystem disorder of unknown aetiology which may have several presentations. The current classification is based on the distribution of skin involvement; if scleroderma is limited to the face and skin distal to the elbows and knees, the disease is classified as limited cutaneous systemic sclerosis (LcSSc). If skin involvement is more extensive it is classified as diffuse cutaneous systemic sclerosis (DcSSc) (LeRoy et al., 1988). Rarely, a diagnosis can be made in the absence of skin involvement; so called scleroderma sine scleroderma. The previously described CREST (calcinosis, Raynaud's phenomenon, oesophageal dysmotility, sclerodactyly, and telangiectasia) syndrome is no longer felt to be a useful diagnostic category, as patients with either LcSSc or DcSSc may have these clinical features (Hachulla et al., 2010).

LcSSc is characterized by Raynaud's phenomenon, which usually precedes other symptoms by several years. The Raynaud's

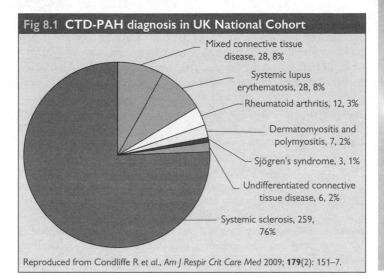

Fig 8.1 **CTD-PAH** diagnosis in UK National Cohort

Mixed connective tissue disease, 28, 8%

Systemic lupus erythematosis, 28, 8%

Rheumatoid arthritis, 12, 3%

Dermatomyositis and polymyositis, 7, 2%

Sjögren's syndrome, 3, 1%

Undifferentiated connective tissue disease, 6, 2%

Systemic sclerosis, 259, 76%

Reproduced from Condliffe R et al., *Am J Respir Crit Care Med* 2009; **179**(2): 151–7.

phenomenon may be severe and may cause digital ulcers or necrosis. It is associated with anti-nuclear antibodies (ANA), which stain in an anti-centromere pattern (Nihtyanova et al., 2010a). Digital capillaroscopy usually reveals tortuous, dilated capillaries, which may help to distinguish these patients from the more common primary Raynaud's phenomenon. Skin thickening usually begins on the fingers (sclerodactyly) and around the mouth and nose.

DcSSc, on the other hand, has a more sudden onset and rapidly progressive course. It is classically associated with anti-topoisomerase-1 antibodies (ATA, also known as anti-Scleroderma-70). Patients with diffuse disease are rarely ACA positive, 70% are either ATA or anti-RNA polymerase antibody positive (Nihtyanova, 2010a). Most internal organ complications are more common in patients with diffuse disease, and these tend to occur in the first three years. After this period, major organ complications are less likely and skin often improves.

Of all the organ involved in SSc patients most frequently suffer with gastrointestinal manifestations. Upper gastrointestinal involvement leads to dysphagia and reflux and, in severe cases, early satiety and post-prandial vomiting. Bacterial overgrowth frequently leads to chronic diarrhoea. Colonic dysmotility may cause constipation and the anal sphincter is often affected leading to faecal incontinence (Forbes & Marie, 2009). Telangiectasia are not restricted to the skin and have been found in mucosa along the entire gastrointestinal tract. In particular gastric antral vascular ectasia (GAVE) or watermelon stomach can produce profound gastrointestinal haemorrhage.

Renal crisis occurs in about 15% of DcSSc, and 5% of LcSSc, and is characterized by an abrupt onset of renal failure and severe hypertension. About 25% of patients require long term dialysis (Denton et al., 2009). Interstitial lung disease occurs in about 38% of DcSSc and 16% of LcSSC within 5 years after the first non-Raynaud's symptoms of SSc. Two randomized controlled trials suggest immunosuppression with cyclophosphamide may have a role in treatment of scleroderma associated interstitial lung disease, although the benefits were limited (Wells et al., 2009). Cardiac involvement may be dramatic with myocarditis, dilated cardiomyopathy and restrictive cardiomyopathy but fortunately remains uncommon as a significant clinical manifestation (around 1%) (Nihtyanova et al., 2010b). Pulmonary hypertension occurs in around 10%, with a possible bias toward limited disease. It may be difficult to recognize in patients with systemic sclerosis because dyspnoea may be caused by many other causes, including anaemia, deconditioning, interstitial lung disease, left ventricular diastolic dysfunction among others (Hachulla et al., 2009b).

Outcomes in SSc are determined by the pattern of organ involvement. There is some evidence that annual internal organ assessments with lung function tests, echocardiography and renal function tests are associated with increased survival (Nihtyanova, 2010b). Auto-antibodies may predict disease pattern or presence of overlap CTDs, e.g. Sjögren's or polymyositis which makes them useful in assessment. Auto-antibody types identified in SSc and overlap syndromes include anti-: topoisomerase, centromere, RNA polymerase, fibrillarin (U3RNP), Th/To, U1RNP, PM-Scl, Ro, La, Ku, SL, XR, double-stranded DNA (dsDNA), fibrillin-1, endothelial cell, matrix metalloproteinases 1 and 3, non-steroidal anti-inflammatory drug-activated gene (Nag-2) and platelet derived growth factor receptor (PDGFR) (Gabrielli et al., 2009). In addition anti-Sm, anti-phospholipid antibodies may be seen in SLE, therefore a wide range of antibody types should be tested in someone presenting with apparent idiopathic PAH. It should be noted that up to 11% of SSc patients may test negative for ANA and around a quarter have no specific antibody subtype (Nihtyanova, 2010a).

Optimally managing this complex disease requires close collaboration between rheumatologists and pulmonary hypertension physicians and as detailed below the approach to managing the pulmonary hypertension is somewhat more nuanced. So a thorough examination for the clinical features of scleroderma, and a screening antibody profile should be performed at diagnosis of PAH. Digital capillaroscopy should also be performed particularly if a history of Raynaud's is elicited.

### 8.3.2 Systemic lupus erythematosus

Systemic lupus erythematosus (SLE) is a cryptogenic condition. Patients usually suffer from constitutional symptoms including: fatigue, hair loss, rash and arthralgias. Indicators of disease activity include an increase in constitutional symptoms, a raised ESR with a relatively low C-reactive protein, low complement levels, lymphopaenia and sometimes other cytopaenias and a rise in anti-dsDNA titres. Nearly all patients with SLE are ANA positive. Anti-Sm and anti-dsDNA antibodies are very specific for SLE but are found in only about 40% of patients. In addition, many have anti-Ro and anti-La antibodies, which are associated with Sjögren's syndrome overlap. 1–2% of pregnancies in women with anti-Ro antibodies may be complicated by foetal heart block and these women need careful surveillance.

Organ complications in SLE are myriad but every clinician treating patients with SLE must be aware of several important complications:

- Neuropsychiatric lupus can mimic almost any neurological condition. It may present insidiously with difficulty in concentrating, headache, memory loss or personality change or more dramatically with seizures, stroke, reduced consciousness, transverse myelitis or peripheral neuropathy. The clinician should be alert for any new neurological symptoms and investigate them carefully (Muscal & Brey, 2010).

- Lupus hepatitis is common and in some patients rises in liver transaminases reflect SLE disease activity. About 20% of patients with SLE have abnormal liver enzyme levels at some point in their illness (Youssef & Tavill, 2002). It is important to consider this in patients treated with hepatotoxic medications.

- Haematological involvement in SLE is multifactorial. There is commonly anaemia of chronic disease. In addition hypoplastic cytopaenias are seen in association with disease activity. This usually affects lymphocytes first, and then other cell lines. There may also be autoimmune haemolytic anaemia, autoimmune thrombocytopaenia and autoimmune leucopaenia, which can be severe (Keeling & Isenberg, 1993).

- Lupus nephritis is a major complication of SLE and screening of every patient with a urine dipstick and blood pressure measurement should occur at each clinic visit. The presence of new hypertension or of blood or protein in the urine should prompt further investigation.

- Pulmonary complications include pneumonia, especially if the patient is on immunosuppressive treatment, interstitial lung disease, pleural effusion and pulmonary emboli, especially in patients with anti-phospholipid antibodies.

The shrinking lung syndrome is thought to be due to weakness of the diaphgram.

• Cardiac complications are less common, but they can include pericarditis and pericardial effusion, myocarditis, Libman-Sacks endocarditis, myocardial infarction and arrhythmias (Doria et al., 2005).

Patients with anti-phospholipid antibodies merit special consideration. There is an overlap between SLE and the anti-phospholipid syndrome. Patients with SLE may make anti-phospholipid antibodies and lupus anticoagulant factors intermittently. These patients are at increased risk of atherosclerotic events, venous and arterial thromboses and developing pulmonary hypertension. Thromboembolic disease is certainly more common in patients with SLE at postmortem (Quadrelli et al., 2009), and the presence of lupus anticoagulant or anti-phospholipid antibodies is associated with a more than four-fold increase in the risk of chronic thromboembolic pulmonary hypertension (Bonderman et al., 2009). This has led to calls to screen SLE patients with lupus anticoagulant or those planning to conceive for pulmonary hypertension (Bijl et al., 2009, Cefle et al., 2009). There are no guidelines on when patients with SLE should be screened for pulmonary hypertension. Symptoms may be difficult to assess as there are so many causes of dyspnoea in SLE: marked fatigue, anaemia, autoimmune thyroid disease, myositis as well as the many respiratory and cardiac complications. There are also several potential causes of pulmonary hypertension in SLE, including recurrent thromboemboli, pulmonary vasculitis, interstitial lung disease, left ventricular disease as well as PAH. There is some evidence that endothelin levels are elevated in patients with SLE and this may contribute to PAH (Pope, 2008).

There may be an important role for immunosuppression with cyclophosphamide and prednisolone in the treatment of PAH associated with SLE and MCTD. This is on the basis of a small, randomized open label study comparing cyclophosphamide to enalapril. This found a treatment benefit in terms of haemodynamic and functional class improvement (Gonzalez-Lopez et al., 2004). A small French retrospective case series suggested that half of patients with SLE or MCTD and PAH respond to immunosuppression with steroids and monthly intravenous cyclophosphamide, especially those with functional class I or II (Sanchez et al., 2006, Jais et al., 2008). Only a few patients with SLE-PAH have been included in the clinical trials of advanced therapies for pulmonary hypertension, although Bosentan was found to be helpful in a small case series (Mok et al., 2007).

The prognosis of patients with SLE-PAH appears to be intermediate between idiopathic PAH and SSc associated PAH. In the UK national pulmonary hypertension data, 1 and 3 year survival in the 28 patients with SLE-PAH were 78% and 74% respectively. Of patients with SLE 75% were treated with advanced therapy whereas 86% received immunosuppression (Condliffe et al., 2009).

### 8.3.3 Mixed connective tissue disease

Mixed connective tissue disease (MCTD) was first described in 1972. It is a syndrome with features of SSc, SLE and polymyositis associated with antibody against U1RNP (ribonuclear protein component of the spliceosome). Patients frequently suffer from Raynaud's, swollen hands, sclerodactyly, arthritis and interstitial lung disease (Venables, 2006). Some investigators feel that with long term follow up, patients usually manifest as SSc, SLE or RA within 5 years (van den Hoogen et al., 1994). Others however feel that the MCTD diagnosis is stable (Frandsen et al., 1996). Pulmonary hypertension is a feared complication, but there is little robust data regarding incidence or response to treatment (Lundberg, 2005).

Confusingly for the non-rheumatologist terms such as undifferentiated connective tissue disease and overlap syndrome exist in the literature. These are often used when patients have features of two or more CTDs including SLE and SSc, e.g. SLE/SSc overlap syndrome.

### 8.3.4 Polymyositis and dermatomyositis

Patients with polymyositis may present with muscle pain and weakness, and are sometimes systemically unwell. Dermatomyositis may present in addition with characteristic rashes (Dalakas et al., 2003). Pulmonary hypertension is a rare complication (Minai, 2009), accounting for 4% of the CTD-PAH cases seen in the UK (Battle et al., 1996).

### 8.3.5 Rheumatoid arthritis

PAH associated with rheumatoid arthritis (RA) is very rare. Given that the prevalence of rheumatoid arthritis in the UK is about 1% (Symmons et al., 2002), and that the prevalence of PAH is about 50 cases per million population (Peacock et al., 2007) any associations may be due to chance and not a true disease association. The anti-cyclic citrullinated peptide antibody is very specific for RA, rheumatoid factor is typically very elevated but lacks predictive value.

### 8.3.6 Sjögren's syndrome

Sjögren's syndrome (SS) is an idiopathic inflammatory disease characterized by dry eyes and dry mouth, due to lymphocytic infiltration of the salivary glands, and autoimmune antibodies, especially anti-Ro and anti-La. It is often seen in conjunction with other CTDs when it is usually termed secondary Sjögren's, but sometimes its presence leads to the term overlap CTD or syndrome. The term primary Sjögren's syndrome is used when it occurs in isolation. Pulmonary hypertension has been reported in the absence of lung disease although interstitial lung disease does occur (Launay et al., 2007). Other associations of SS are peripheral neuropathy, thrombocyto-paenia, leucopaenia, peripheral neuropathy, lymphoma and vasculitis (Ramos-Casals et al., 2008).

## 8.4 Treatments used in connective tissue diseases

Patients with connective tissue disease are frequently treated with immunosuppression. The most widely used and rapidly acting immu-nosuppressants are corticosteroids. Side effects of corticosteroids limit long term use at a high dose, and so steroid sparing agents are used. Cyclophosphamide is the most potent immunosuppres-sive agent but is associated with bladder cancer, loss of fertility, alo-pecia and cytopaenias. Its use is reserved for severe disease such as lupus nephritis, scleroderma lung disease and severe vasculitis. Other drugs such as azathioprine, methotrexate, and mycopheno-late mofetil are used for a wide range of indications. They require regular blood monitoring for cytopaenias and hepatotoxicity. In the event of intercurrent infection, chronic steroid treatment must be increased, but most other immunosuppressants should be stopped abruptly.

## 8.5 Pathophysiology of CTD PAH

Part of the difficulty with CTD patients is the number of poten-tial mechanisms by which pulmonary hypertension might develop. These are not mutually exclusive so, theoretically, a patient with CTD could have true PAH, left heart disease (from hypertension or myocarditis), hypoxia (secondary to interstitial lung disease) and pulmonary thromboemboli (from anti-phospholipid syndrome). A discussion of the current diagnostic classification of pulmonary hypertension can be found in the current European and American guidelines (Simonneau et al., 2009, Galie et al., 2009a).

The different disease associations and types of PAH are linked because they share pathophysiological features. In the simplest terms small, distal pulmonary arterioles become constricted and undergo abnormal vascular remodelling. This creates the increased pulmonary vascular resistance seen on haemodynamic studies. Some of these features are common to scleroderma and associated organ damage. These similarities have helped to drive our understanding of PAH and develop therapies.

The early vascular lesion in scleroderma affects small vessels causing endothelial cell injury (Prescott et al., 1992). This leads to vasoconstriction, apoptosis, increased cell adhesion molecule expression, a pro-coagulant state, recruitment of inflammatory cells to the perivascular space, promotion of vascular smooth muscle cell proliferation and dysregulation of vasculogenesis (Gabrielli et al., 2009). Pericytes and vascular smooth muscle cells proliferate vigorously resulting in increased vascular wall thickness. These changes are analogous to several of the hallmarks of histopathological changes in PAH: medial hypertrophy, intimal proliferation, adventitial thickening with perivascular inflammatory cell infiltration and thrombotic lesions (Dorfmuller et al., 2007). Mononuclear T cells and B cells are seen around the plexiform lesions in PAH and in SSc skin samples.

In scleroderma progression from the inflammatory phase to fibrosis is driven by fibroblast orchestrated collagen deposition analogous to neo-intimal remodelling in PAH (Gabrielli et al., 2009). This accumulation of extra-cellular matrix and collagen disrupts tissue architecture. These processes combined lead to the reduced number of small vessels seen in later stages of SSc as they are obliterated without compensation via angiogenesis. The complex dilated and plexiform lesions seen in late PAH are thought to be due to aberrant channels formed as a result of abnormal endothelial cell proliferation (Tuder et al., 1994). The pattern of vasculopathy in SScPAH has been examined in light of the poor response to therapy and survival seen. When compared with idiopathic PAH, SScPAH lung tissue shows more frequent fibrosis of venules with capillary congestion and fewer plexiform lesions (Overbeek et al., 2009). This pattern of involvement is similar in some respects to pulmonary veno-occlusive disease, a subtype of PAH with a poor prognosis.

Although expression of the cytokines TGF-β (transforming growth factor) and CTGF (connective tissue growth factor) is enhanced in scleroderma, genetic mutations of the upstream bone morphogenetic protein receptor 2 (BMPR2) found in idiopathic and heritable PAH have not been seen in SScPAH. Gene association studies of the TGF-β superfamily member, have found a polymorphism in SScPAH for the endoglin (ENG) gene otherwise associated with hereditary haemorrhagic telangiectasia (Wipff et al., 2007). Many more candidate genes have been found which relate to inflammatory pathways in SSc.

The presence of ANA, rheumatoid factor, immunoglobulin G and complement fraction deposits in small vessel walls suggest an autoimmune process driving a pulmonary vasculopathy in SScPAH. In particular anti-endothelial cell antibodies seen in the serum of 40–50% of SSc patients cause endothelial cell injury (Gabrielli et al., 2009).

The detection of further auto-antibodies to fibroblasts (Tamby et al., 2006) and increased interleukin-1 and -6 support this theory, but many of these features are also seen in idiopathic PAH. The response of a subgroup of patients with MCTD or SLE associated PAH to immunosuppressive therapy has been used as further evidence of the role of inflammation although there are no reports of such a response in SScPAH (Venables, 2006). Platelet-derived growth factor (PDGF) is another mediator implicated in PAH and SSc. The PDGF receptor is over-expressed in smooth muscle and can be stimulated by auto-antibodies. PDGF promotes pericyte to fibroblast transition and inhibiting agents are being trialled for PAH and SSc.

Endothelial dysfunction results in persistent reduction of nitric oxide and prostacyclin levels with increased thromboxane A2 and endothelin-1 levels. Prostacyclin has been utilized in therapy for digital ischaemia in SSc. Deficiency prevents cyclic AMP formation and thereby increases smooth muscle cell proliferation and platelet aggregation. Endothelin-1 is a potent vasoconstrictor, mitogen pro-fibrotic and pro-inflammatory molecule. Blockade of endothelin-1 receptors has been shown to be effective in digital ulcers in SSc. Selective serotonin (5-HT) reuptake inhibitors are helpful for Raynaud's. The many different 5-HT receptors have made it difficult to develop a therapy that targets the lungs without causing many side effects.

A low diffusing capacity for carbon monoxide (DLco) has been shown to be predictive of the development of PH in scleroderma (Steen & Medsger, 2003). Recently DLco and high NT-proBNP levels have been shown to be independent predictors of PAH which can be used in conjunction (Allanore et al., 2008). In comparison with idiopathic PAH, patients with SScPAH have lower values for DLco even though total lung capacity is not reduced significantly (Kawut et al., 2003, Fisher et al., 2006). At the same time idiopathic PAH patients had higher mean PA pressures and PVR but significantly better survival (Overbeek et al., 2008). This higher mortality has led to consideration of the state of the right ventricle in CTDPAH. Certainly N-terminal pro B-type natriuretic peptide is a useful biomarker for CTDPAH, but attempts to replicate this value in idiopathic PAH have been less consistent, possibly because the right ventricle works more effectively in idiopathic PAH (Mathai et al., 2009). Cardiac MRI studies have found a high prevalence of abnormalities in SSc patients including right ventricle dilation in the absence of PAH (Hachulla et al., 2009c). Applying a haemodynamic approach a reduction in right ventricle contractility can be demonstrated in SScPAH compared with idiopathic PAH (Overbeek et al., 2008). This would be consistent with the poor exercise capacity and survival outcomes seen in SSc.

## 8.5.1 Treatment of CTD PAH

Standard therapies for right heart failure, such as diuretics and digoxin, can be applied to CTDPAH patients, with consideration for other issues related to CTD. Oxygen therapy can be helpful, particularly in patients with significant interstitial lung disease associated with CTD. If not already in use then assessment should be undertaken, ideally including nocturnal and ambulatory requirements. Anticoagulation with coumarin agents has been shown to be beneficial in idiopathic, heritable and anorexigen induced PAH and the rationale for therapy is the same in CTDPAH (reducing pulmonary intravascular thrombosis) (Galie et al., 2009a) However, the presence of anaemia or a bleeding diathesis, such as the GAVE syndrome, may preclude such treatment. Limited evidence exists for immunosuppressive agents, a subgroup of MCTD and SLE patients may exhibit good treatment response (Venables, 2006). Calcium channel blockers are useful for Raynaud's rather than PAH in CTD patients. Haemodynamic response to vasodilator challenge is rare and survival seems to be unaffected by this phenomenon (Galie et al., 2009a).

Improved understanding of the pathobiology of PAH has led to the development of new therapies that have significantly improved symptoms and survival for people with PAH, including those with CTD (Williams et al., 2006). Randomized clinical trials have shown that three groups of agents are beneficial these include 1) the endothelin receptor antagonists (ERA): bosentan, ambrisentan and sitaxentan, 2) the phosphodiesterase type 5 inhibitors (PDE-5I): sildenafil and tadalafil, and 3) the prostanoids: epoprostenol, treprostinil (not licensed in the UK), and iloprost (Ito et al., 2007). The majority of patients in all but one of the clinical trials are idiopathic PAH patients and the amount of data relating to CTDPAH differs from treatment to treatment.

The only therapy that has been specifically evaluated in a multicentre randomized controlled trial in CTDPAH is intravenous epoprostenol. In a population with SScPAH the primary endpoint, 6-minute walk distance was significantly improved at 12 weeks in the 56 patients treated with epoprostenol compared with 55 patients that received conventional therapy alone (median treatment effect +108 m), and significant improvements were observed in a number of haemodynamic endpoints (Badesch et al., 2000). Despite this success, follow up registries failed to show a clear improvement in survival (Ito et al., 2007, Overbeek et al., 2009).

Assessing the efficacy of other prostanoids in the CTD population is difficult, this appears to range from apparently no benefit with oral beraprost (Galie et al., 2002, Barst et al., 2003), to consistent with the impact observed in idiopathic PAH but not reaching significance with inhaled iloprost in the AIR trial (Olschewski et al., 2002), to some significant benefits in the subpopulation of 90 patients with CTDPAH in the subcutaneous treprostinil trial (Simonneau et al., 2002). Unfortunately, the mixed population in the treprostinil trial (25 patients with DcSSc, 20 LcSSc patients, 25 cases of SLE, and 20 patients diagnosed with MCTD/overlap syndroms) makes it difficult to know if the SSc population benefited.

The most extensive data on the treatment of CTDPAH is found in trials and registries with endothelin receptor antagonists, however, even here the situation remains confused. 99 patients with CTDPAH were included in three pivotal trials with bosentan, of these 66 had SScPAH (Channick et al., 2001, Rubin et al., 2002, Galie et al., 2007). The response to therapy of the CTDPAH sub group was consistent with the overall study population (similar in magnitude and direction), but no significant changes were observed. A prospective open label study (TRUST) of bosentan in CTDPAH reported improvement in functional class and 92% survival at 48 weeks (Denton et al., 2008). Follow up registry data in both SScPAH (Tuder et al., 1994) and CTDPAH (Pope et al., 2007) show that survival is significantly improved when compared to historical data.

Sitaxentan (an endothelin receptor A specific antagonist) has been studied in three double blind trials (Barst et al., 2004, Langleben et al., 2004, Oudiz, 2006). In the individual trials there was no statistically significant difference on six minute walking distance in the subpopulation with CTD. However, the 6-minute walk test showed an improvement of 20 to 25 m for the CTD population. Post hoc analysis has been undertaken on the 119 patients with CTDPAH allocated to the effective dose (100 mg), 58 of whom received placebo and 61 treated (Siebold, 2005). On active therapy 6-minute walk distance increased by 25m, giving a net benefit over placebo of 38 m (P = 0.007). Post-hoc analysis of the open-label follow up of the STRIDE 2X trial, suggested a significant prognostic benefit for sitaxentan over bosentan (Highland et al., 2006), though survival at 2 years was identical to that published for the bosentan treated populations.

Ambrisentan has been evaluated in 2 randomized controlled multi-centre studies which included 124 patients with CTDPAH (80% scleroderma or mixed connective tissue disease), 6MWD improved by nearly 20 m in the 5 & 10mg groups (net benefit over placebo 26m (p = ns) (Galie et al., 2008). Data on file from the 2 year extension study indicates that the rate of clinical worsening for the CTD population was almost identical to that of the total population (GlaxoSmithKline AMB 029 & 037).

Two phosphodiesterase-5 inhibitors have completed pivotal trials in PAH. In the Super trial 62 patients with CTDPAH were randomized to one of the three treatment arms. The direction and magnitude of benefit was similar to the overall trial effect, but not significant because of population size (Galie et al., 2005). In the Phirst trial, 95 CTDPAH patients were randomized to each of the three tadalafil treatment arms or placebo, similar improvements in 6-minute walk distance and time to clinical worsening were observed, again not reaching significance in the sub group (Galie et al., 2009b).

As the largest subgroup the bulk of published data deals with SScPAH. PAH-specific therapy during the era of monotherapy (2001–2006) improved the prognosis for patients with PAH associated with SSc, the 3-year survival is 67% for patients in World Health Organization functional classes (WHO FC) I/II, decreasing to 48% for WHO FC III and 21% for WHO FC IV patients with SSc (Condliffe et al., 2009).

## 8.6 Combination therapy

While the evidence base for monotherapy is far from satisfactory it is evident that the magnitude and direction of efficacy is similar in the CTDPAH subgroups and it is clear that the most recalcitrant group (SSc associated PAH) has benefited through improved survival in all registries of oral therapies. The focus of clinical investigation has now moved to combination therapy, and is gradually shifting toward time to clinical worsening as the more important endpoint. Unfortunately, to date the trend for including relatively small numbers of CTDPAH patients and not performing prespecified analysis of this subgroup continues.

In the PACES-1 trial of sildenafil added to epoprostenol 45 patients had CTDPAH (31 with SSc)—the dominant benefit in terms of reducing mortality was seen in those with a 6-minute walk distance of less than 325 m (Simonneau et al., 2008). This is where one finds the bulk of the CTDPAH population and this has tended to be the population with the greatest contribution to clinical events, it is conceivable that this subpopulation will become a significant contributor to improved outcome as the primary endpoint shifts to time to clinical worsening.

## 8.7 The future of CTD PAH

CTDPAH is coming of age. We now understand that not all types of CTDPAH have the same prognosis, the bulk of data indicate that the event rate remains high in this population despite therapy and that 6-minute walk distance as a primary endpoint has disadvantaged this group. There is good but far from conclusive evidence that the prognosis of this population has been substantially improved by ERA therapy and weaker evidence for PDE 5 inhibitors. The range of confounders in this population is also now better described, thus the data necessary to determine if an event is due to worsening of PAH rather than associated multisystem disease activity is now clear. As we move toward an era of trials with time to clinical worsening as the primary endpoint, the advantages of including substantial numbers of patients with CTDPAH will become increasingly evident, and pre-specified subgroup analysis of the CTDPAH population mandatory.

# References

Allanore Y, Borderie D, Avouac J et al. (2008) High N-terminal pro-brain natriuretic peptide levels and low diffusing capacity for carbon monoxide as independent predictors of the occurrence of precapillary pulmonary arterial hypertension in patients with systemic sclerosis. *Arthritis Rheum* **58**(1): 284–91.

Alpert MA, Goldberg SH, Singsen BH et al. (1983) Cardiovascular manifestations of mixed connective tissue disease in adults. *Circulation* **68**(6): 1182–93.

Badesch DB, Tapson VF, McGoon MD et al. (2000) Continuous intravenous epoprostenol for pulmonary hypertension due to the scleroderma spectrum of disease. A randomized, controlled trial. *Ann Intern Med* **132**(6): 425–34.

Barst RJ, McGoon M, McLaughlin V et al. (2003) Beraprost therapy for pulmonary arterial hypertension. *J Am Coll Cardiol* **41**(12): 2119–25.

Barst RJ, Langleben D, Frost A et al. (2004) Sitaxentan therapy for pulmonary arterial hypertension. *Am J Respir Crit Care Med* **169**: 441–7.

Battle RW, Davitt MA, Cooper SM, Buckley LM, Leib ES, Beglin PA et al. (1996) Prevalence of pulmonary hypertension in limited and diffuse scleroderma. *Chest* **110**: 1515–9.

Bijl M, Bootsma H, Kallenberg CG (2009) Pulmonary arterial hypertension in systemic lupus erythematosus: should we bother? *Rheumatology (Oxford)* **48**(12): 1471–2.

Bonderman D, Wilkens H, Wakounig S et al. (2009) Risk factors for chronic thromboembolic pulmonary hypertension. *Eur Respir J* **33**(2): 325–31.

Cefle A, Inanc M, Sayarlioglu M et al. (2009) Pulmonary hypertension in systemic lupus erythematosus: relationship with antiphospholipid antibodies and severe disease outcome. *Rheumatol Int.* [Epub ahead of print].

Channick RN, Simonneau G, Sitbon O et al. (2001) Effects of the dual endothelin-receptor antagonist bosentan in patients with pulmonary hypertension: a randomised placebo-controlled study. *Lancet* **358**(9288): 1119–23.

Condliffe R, Kiely DG, Peacock AJ et al. (2009) Connective tissue disease-associated pulmonary arterial hypertension in the modern treatment era. *Am J Respir Crit Care Med* **179**(2): 151–7.

Dalakas MC, Hohlfeld R (2003) Polymyositis and dermatomyositis. *Lancet* **362**(9388): 971–82.

Data on file GlaxoSmithKline AMB 029 & 037.

Dawson JK, Goodson NG, Graham DR, Lynch MP (2000) Raised pulmonary artery pressures measured with Doppler echocardiography in rheumatoid arthritis patients. *Rheumatology (Oxford)* **39**(12): 1320–5.

Denton CP, Pope JE, Peter HH *et al.* on behalf of the TRacleer Use in PAH associated with Scleroderma and Connective Tissue Diseases (TRUST) Investigators (2008) Long-term effects of bosentan on quality of life, survival, safety and tolerability in pulmonary arterial hypertension related to connective tissue diseases. *Ann Rheum Dis* **67**: 1222–8.

Denton CP, Lapadula G, Mouthon L, Müller-Ladner U (2009) Renal complications and scleroderma renal crisis. *Rheumatology (Oxford)* 2009;**48** Suppl 3:iii32-5.

Dorfmüller P, Humbert M, Perros F, Sanchez O, Simonneau G, Müller KM, Capron F (2007) Fibrous remodeling of the pulmonary venous system in pulmonary arterial hypertension associated with connective tissue diseases. *Hum Pathol* 38(6): 893–902. Epub 2007 Mar 21.

Doria A, Iaccarino L, Sarzi-Puttini P, Atzeni F, Turriel M, Petri M (2005) Cardiac involvement in systemic lupus erythematosus. *Lupus* **14**(9): 683–6.

Fisher MR, Mathai SC, Champion HC *et al.* (2006) Clinical differences between idiopathic and scleroderma-related pulmonary hypertension. *Arthritis Rheum* **54**(9): 3043–50.

Forbes A, Marie I (2009) Gastrointestinal complications: the most frequent internal complications of systemic sclerosis. *Rheumatology (Oxford)* **48** Suppl 3: ii36–9.

Frandsen PB, Kriegbaum NJ, Ullman S, Høier-Madsen M, Wiik A, Halberg P (1996) Follow-up of 151 patients with high-titer U1RNP antibodies. *Clin Rheumatol* **15**(3): 254–60.

Gabrielli A, Avvedimento EV, Krieg T. Scleroderma (2009) *N Engl J Med* **360**(19): 1989–2003.

Galiè N, Humbert M, Vachiery JL *et al.* (2002) Effects of beraprost sodium, an oral prostacyclin analogue in patients with pulmonary arterial hypertension: a randomised, double-blind, placebo-controlled trial. *J Am Coll Cardiol* **39**: 1496–502.

Galie N, Ghofrani HA, Torbicki A *et al.* (2005) Sildenafil citrate therapy for pulmonary arterial hypertension. *N Engl J Med* **353**(20): 2148–57.

Galie N, Hoeper MM, Jansa P *et al.* (2007) Bosentan improves hemodynamics and delays time to clinical worsening in patients with mildly symptomatic Pulmonary Arterial Hypertension (PAH): results of the EARLY study. *European Heart Journal* **28**[suppl.1]: 140. 2007. Ref Type: Abstract.

Galiè N, Richards D, Hutchinson T, Dufton C (2008) Ambrisentan therapy for patients with PAH associated with connective tissue disease (PAH-CTD): one year follow-up. European Respiratory Society Annual Congress Berlin 2008 Abstract E1418.

Galiè N, Hoeper MM, Humbert M *et al.* (2009a) Guidelines for the diagnosis and treatment of pulmonary hypertension: The Task Force for the Diagnosis and Treatment of Pulmonary Hypertension of the European Society of Cardiology (ESC) and the European Respiratory Society (ERS), endorsed by the International Society of Heart and Lung Transplantation (ISHLT). *Eur Heart J* **30**(20): 2493–2537.

Galiè N, Brundage BH, Ghofrani HA *et al.* (2009b) Tadalafil therapy for pulmonary arterial hypertension. *Circulation* **119**(22): 2894–903.

Ghofrani A for the Sildenafil 1140 study group (2004) Efficacy and safety of sildenafil in pulmonary arterial hypertension: results of a multinational randomized, double blind placebo controlled trial. Americal College of Chest Physicians.

Gonzalez-Lopez L, Cardona-Muñoz EG, Celis A *et al.* (2004) Therapy with intermittent pulse cyclophosphamide for pulmonary hypertension associated with systemic lupus erythematosus. *Lupus* **13**(2): 105–12.

Hachulla E, Gressin V, Guillevin L *et al.* (2005) Early detection of pulmonary arterial hypertension in systemic sclerosis: a French nationwide prospective multicenter study. *Arthritis Rheum* **52**: 3792–800.

Hachulla E, de Groote P, Gressin V *et al.* (2009a) The three-year incidence of pulmonary arterial hypertension associated with systemic sclerosis in a multicenter nationwide longitudinal study in France. *Arthritis Rheum* **60**(6): 1831–9.

Hachulla E, Bervar JF, Launay D *et al.* (2009b) [Dyspnea upon exertion in systemic scleroderma: from symptom to etiological diagnosis] *Presse Med* **38**(6): 911–26. [Article in French]

Hachulla AL, Launay D, Gaxotte V *et al.* (2009c) Cardiac magnetic resonance imaging in systemic sclerosis: a cross-sectional observational study of 52 patients. *Ann Rheum Dis* **68**(12): 1878–84. Epub 2008 Dec 3.

Hachulla E, Launay D (2010) Diagnosis and Classification of Systemic Sclerosis. *Clin Rev Allergy Immunol* 2010 Feb 10. [Epub ahead of print].

Highland KB, Strange C, Girgis RE, Black C (2006) Comparison of sitaxentan and bosentan in pulmonary arterial hypertension associated with connective tissue disease [abstract]. *Ann Rheum Dis* **65**(Suppl II): 393.

Humbert M (2005) Post marketing surveillance survey of use of Bosentan in pulmonary arterial hypertension., oral presentation ATS annual meeting.

Hunzelmann N, Genth E, Krieg T *et al.* Registry of the German Network for Systemic Scleroderma (2008) The registry of the German Network for Systemic Scleroderma: frequency of disease subsets and patterns of organ involvement. *Rheumatology (Oxford).* **47**(8): 1185–92.

Ito T, Ozawa K, Shimada K (2007) Current drug targets and future therapy of pulmonary arterial hypertension. *Curr Med Chem* **14**(6): 719–33.

Jais X, Launay D, Yaici A *et al.* (2008) Immunosuppressive therapy in lupus- and mixed connective tissue disease-associated pulmonary arterial hypertension: a retrospective analysis of twenty-three cases. *Arthritis Rheum* **58**(2): 521–31.

Kawut SM, Taichman DB, Archer-Chicko CL, Palevsky HI, Kimmel SE (2003) Hemodynamics and survival in patients with pulmonary arterial hypertension related to systemic sclerosis. *Chest* **123**(2): 344–50.

Keeling DM, Isenberg DA (1993) Haematological manifestations of systemic lupus erythematosus. *Blood Rev* **7**(4): 199–207.

Langleben D, Brock T, Dixon R, Barst R (2004) STRIDE 1: Effects of the selective ETA receptor antagonist, sitaxentan sodium, in a patient population with pulmonary arterial hypertension that meets traditional inclusion criteria of previous pulmonary arterial hypertension trials. *J Cardiovasc Pharmacol* **44**: S80–S84.

Launay D, Hachulla E, Hatron PY, Jais X, Simonneau G, Humbert M (2007) Pulmonary arterial hypertension: a rare complication of primary Sjögren syndrome: report of 9 new cases and review of the literature. *Medicine (Baltimore)* **86**(5): 299–315.

LeRoy EC, Black C, Fleischmajer R *et al.* (1988) Scleroderma (systemic sclerosis): classification, subsets, and pathogenesis. *J Rheumatol* **15**: 202.

Li EK, Tam LS (1999) Pulmonary hypertension in systemic lupus erythematosus: clinical association and survival in 18 patients. *J Rheumatol* **26**(9): 1923–9.

Lundberg IE (2005) The prognosis of mixed connective tissue disease. *Rheum Dis Clin North Am* **31**(3): 535–47, vii–viii.

Marasini B, Massarotti M, Cossutta R *et al.* (2005) Pulmonary Hypertension in Autoimmune rheumatic diseases. *Rheumatismo* **57**: 114–8.

Mathai SC, Bueso M, Hummers LK *et al.* (2009) Disproportionate elevation og NT-proBNP in scleroderma-related pulmonary hypertension. *Eur Respir J* **35**(1): 95–104. Epub 2009 Jul 30.

McLaughlin VV, Archer SL, Badesch DB *et al.* (2009) ACCF/AHA 2009 expert consensus document on pulmonary hypertension a report of the American College of Cardiology Foundation Task Force on Expert Consensus Documents and the American Heart Association developed in collaboration with the American College of Chest Physicians; American Thoracic Society, Inc.; and the Pulmonary Hypertension Association. *J Am Coll Cardiol* **53**(17): 1573–1619.

Michels H (1997) Course of mixed connective tissue disease in children. *Ann Med* **29**(5): 359–64.

Minai OA (2009) Pulmonary hypertension in polymyositis-dermatomyositis: clinical and hemodynamic characteristics and response to vasoactive therapy. *Lupus* **18**(11): 1006–10.

Mok MY, Tsang PL, Lam YM, Lo Y, Wong WS, Lau CS (2007) Bosentan use in systemic lupus erythematosus patients with pulmonary arterial hypertension. *Lupus* **16**(4): 279–85.

Mukerjee D, St George D, Coleiro B *et al.* (2003) Prevalence and outcome in systemic sclerosis associated pulmonary arterial hypertension: application of a registry approach. *Ann Rheum Dis* **62**(11): 1088–93.

Mukerjee D, St. George D, Knight C *et al.* (2004) Echocardiography and pulmonary function as screening tests for pulmonary arterial hypertension in systemic sclerosis. *Rheumatology* **43**(4): 461–6.

Muscal E, Brey RL (2010) Neurologic manifestations of systemic lupus erythematosus in children and adults. *Neurol Clin* **28**(1): 61–73.

Nihtyanova SI, Denton CP (2010a) Autoantibodies as predictive tools in systemic sclerosis. *Nat Rev Rheumatol* **6**(2): 112–6.

Nihtyanova SI, Tang EC, Coghlan JG, Wells AU, Black CM, Denton CP (2010b) Improved survival in systemic sclerosis is associated with better ascertainment of internal organ disease: a retrospective cohort study. *QJM* **103**(2): 109–15.

117

Olschewski H, Simonneau G, Galiè N, Higenbottam T, Naeije R, Rubin LJ (2002) Inhaled iloprost for severe pulmonary hypertension. *N Engl J Med* **347**: 322–9.

Oudiz R (2006) Functional Class Improvement with Sitaxentan in Patients With Class II-IV Pulmonary Arterial Hypertension (PAH). *ATS* May 2006 A824.

Overbeek MJ, Lankhaar JW, Westerhof N *et al*. (2008) Right ventricular contractility in systemic sclerosis-associated and idiopathic pulmonary arterial hypertension. *Eur Respir J* **31**(6): 1160–6. Epub 2008 Jan 23.

Overbeek MJ, Vonk MC, Boonstra A *et al*. (2009) Pulmonary arterial hypertension in limited cutaneous systemic sclerosis: a distinctive vasculopathy. *Eur Respir J* **34**(2): 371-9. Epub 2009 Mar 12.

Pan TL, Thumboo J, Boey ML (2000) Primary and secondary pulmonary hypertension in systemic lupus erythematosus. *Lupus* **9**(5): 338–42.

Peacock AJ, Murphy NF, McMurray JJ, Caballero L, Stewart S (2007) An epidemiological study of pulmonary arterial hypertension. *Eur Respir J* **30**(1): 104–9.

Pope JE, Gabrielli A, Peter H *et al*. (2007) Long-term Effects of Bosentan Treatment on Survival in Patients with Pulmonary Arterial Hypertension (PAH) Related to Connective Tissue Disease (CTD). *Arthritis Rheum* 56 (9 Suppl): 1199.

Pope J (2008) An update in pulmonary hypertension in systemic lupus erythematosus—do we need to know about it? *Lupus* **17**(4): 274–7.

Prabu A, Patel K, Yee CS *et al*. (2009) Prevalence and risk factors for pulmonary arterial hypertension in patients with lupus. *Rheumatology (Oxford)* **48**(12): 1506–11.

Prescott RJ, Freemont AJ, Jones CJ, Hoyland J, Fielding P (1992) Sequential dermal microvascular and perivascular changes in the development of scleroderma. *J Pathol* **166**(3): 255–63.

Quadrelli SA, Alvarez C, Arce SC, Paz L, Sarano J, Sobrino EM, Manni J (2009) Pulmonary involvement of systemic lupus erythematosus: analysis of 90 necropsies. *Lupus* **18**(12): 1053–60.

Ramos-Casals M, Solans R, Rosas J *et al*. GEMESS Study Group (2008) Primary Sjögren syndrome in Spain: clinical and immunologic expression in 1010 patients. *Medicine (Baltimore)* **87**(4): 210–9.

Rubin LJ, Badesch DB, Barst RJ *et al*. (2002) Bosentan therapy for pulmonary arterial hypertension. *N Engl J Med* **346**: 896–903.

Sanchez O, Sitbon O, Jais X, Simonneau G, Humbert M (2006) Immunosuppressive therapy in connective tissue diseases-associated pulmonary arterial hypertension. *Chest* **130**(1): 182–9.

Siebold J (2005) Sitaxentan, a Selective Endothelin-A Receptor Antagonist, Improves Exercise Capacity in Pulmonary Arterial Hypertension (PAH) Associated with Connective Tissue Disease (CTD) *Chest*: A2704.

Seibold JR, Denton CP, Distler O *et al*. (2008) The DETECT study: A two-stage, prospective, observational, cohort study in scleroderma patients to evaluate screening tests and the incidence of pulmonary arterial hypertension and pulmonary hypertension. Presented at ACR 2008.

Simonneau G, Barst RJ, Galiè N et al. (2002) Continuous subcutaneous infusion of treprostinil, a prostacyclin analogue, in patients with pulmonary arterial hypertension: a double-blind, randomised, placebo-controlled trial. *Am J Respir Crit Care Med* **165**: 800–4.

Simonneau G, Rubin LJ, Galiè N et al. (2008) Addition of sildenafil to long-term intravenous epoprostenol therapy in patients with pulmonary arterial hypertension: a randomized trial. *Ann Intern Med* **149**(8): 521-30.

Simonneau G, Robbins IM, Beghetti M et al. (2009) Updated Clinical Classification of Pulmonary Hypertension. *J Am Coll Cardiol* **54**(Supp S): S43–S54.

Steen V, Medsger TA Jr. (2003) Predictors of isolated pulmonary hypertension in patients with systemic sclerosis and limited cutaneous involvement. *Arthritis Rheum* 48(2): 516–22.

Symmons D, Turner G, Webb R et al. (2002) The prevalence of rheumatoid arthritis in the United Kingdom: new estimates for a new century. *Rheumatology (Oxford)* **41**(7): 793-800.

Tamby MC, Humbert M, Guilpain P et al. (2006) Antibodies to fibroblasts in idiopathic and scleroderma-associated pulmonary hypertension. *Eur Respir J* **28**(4): 799–807.

Tanaka E, Harigai M, Tanaka M et al. (2002) Pulmonary hypertension in systemic lupus erythematosus: evaluation of clinical characteristics and response to immunosuppressive treatment. *J Rheumatol* **29**(2): 282–7.

Tuder RM, Groves B, Badesch DB, Voelkel NF (1994) Exuberant endothelial cell growth and elements of inflammation are present in plexiform lesions of pulmonary hypertension. *Am J Pathol* **144**(2): 275–85.

van den Hoogen FH, Spronk PE, Boerbooms AM et al. (1994) Long-term follow-up of 46 patients with anti-(U1)snRNP antibodies. *Br J Rheumatol* **33**(12): 1117–20.

Venables PJ (2006) Mixed connective tissue disease. *Lupus* **15**(3): 132–7.

Vlachoyiannopoulos PG, Dafni UG, Pakas I et al. (2000) Systemic scleroderma in Greece: low mortality and strong linkage with HLA-DRB1*1104 allele. *Ann Rheum Dis* **59**(5): 359–67.

Wells AU, Steen V, Valentini G (2009) Pulmonary complications: one of the most challenging complications of systemic sclerosis. *Rheumatology (Oxford)* **48** Suppl 3: iii40–4.

Wigley F, Mayes M, Lima J et al. (2004) The point prevalence of undiagnosed pulmonary arterial hypertension in patients with connective tissue disease (CTD) attending community based rheumatology clinics (Uncover). ACR annual scientific meeting 2004 presentation no 1057.

Williams MH, Das C, Handler CE et al. (2006) Systemic sclerosis associated pulmonary hypertension: improved survival in the current era. *Heart* **92**(7): 926-32.

Winslow TM, Ossipov MA, Fazio GP et al. (1995) Five year follow up study of the prevalence and progression of pulmonary hypertension in systemic lupus erythematosus. *Am Heart J* **129**: 510–5.

Wipff J, Kahan A, Hachulla E *et al.* (2007) Association between an endo-glin gene polymorphism and systemic sclerosis-related pulmonary arterial hypertension. *Rheumatology (Oxford)* **46**(4): 622–5. Epub 2006 Dec 13.

Yoshida A, Katayama M (2001) Pulmonary Hypertension in Patients with Connective Tissue Diseases. *Nippon Rinsho* **59**(6): 2001–6.

Youssef WI, Tavill AS (2002) Connective tissue diseases and the liver. *J Clin Gastroenterol* **35**(4): 345–9.

## Chapter 9

# Eisenmenger complex

Konstantinos Dimopoulos and
Georgios Giannakoulas

---

**Key points**

- Eisenmenger syndrome differs significantly from other types of pulmonary arterial hypertension in terms of pathophysiology and natural history
- The type and size of the congenital heart defect in Eisenmenger syndrome is important, as it has physiological and prognostic implications
- Eisenmenger syndrome is associated with multiple systemic complications and multiorgan failure
- Advanced therapies have been shown to improve haemodynamics and exercise capacity in Eisenmenger patients. However, supportive measures are as important in the management of these patients.

---

Despite advances in diagnosis and treatment, including surgical repair, of congenital heart disease, 5% to 10% of the total adult population of patients with congenital heart disease (ACHD) develop pulmonary arterial hypertension (PAH). PAH, in turn impacts on quality of life and survival of patients, especially those with near-systemic pulmonary arterial pressures. Improved understanding of the pathophysiology of Eisenmenger syndrome has led to better patient care.

## 9.1 Eisenmenger syndrome: pathophysiology and difference to other forms of PAH

### 9.1.1 Definition

Eisenmenger syndrome is defined as pulmonary hypertension in the presence of reversed or bidirectional shunting. Shunting may occur at different levels and shunts can be divided into pre-tricuspid, i.e. atrial septal defects (ASDs), or post-tricuspid, i.e. non-restrictive ventricular septal defects (VSDs), patent ductus arteriosus (PDA) and aortopulmonary windows.

### 9.1.2 Pathophysiology

The pathophysiology and natural history of Eisenmenger syndrome varies significantly according to the presence of a pre- or post-tricuspid shunt. Most commonly in Eisenmenger patients, a post-tricuspid shunt is present (e.g. VSD, atrioventricular septal defect, PDA, complex cardiac anatomy), with or without an associated pre-tricuspid defect. In these patients, structural alterations of the pulmonary vascular circulation occur in early childhood due to persistent exposure of the pulmonary circulation to increased flow and pressure. These changes are progressive and soon become irreversible (within the first 1–2 years of life) if the defect is not promptly repaired.

Elevated shear stress and circumferential stretch of the pulmonary vascular bed, caused by markedly increased pulmonary blood flow, triggers endothelial dysfunction and vascular remodelling. Typical histologic changes include smooth muscle cell proliferation, increase in extracellular matrix and intravascular thrombosis. Once the increasing pulmonary vascular resistance equals or exceeds systemic resistance, the left-to-right shunt becomes bi-directional or reversed and the development of Eisenmenger syndrome occurs. Irreversible pulmonary arterial hypertension is typically associated with pulmonary vascular resistance values over 800 dyn.s.cm$^{-5}$.

The rate of progression of pulmonary arterial disease, however, varies according to the type and size of the defect. Large (non-restrictive) VSDs and PDAs are more likely to induce an early and more severe pulmonary vascular disease. Patients with pre-tricuspid defects, i.e. large ASDs, can develop PAH, but rarely to systemic levels (Eisenmenger ASD). Occasionally, patients with pre-tricuspid shunts develop severe PAH even after early repair of the defect. Patients with a sinus venosus ASD are also more prone to developing PAH, possibly suggesting the presence of genetic or other predisposing factors in these individuals.

Patients with complex pulmonary atresia and multiple aortopulmonary collaterals may also develop significant PAH. This is often segmental, affecting parts of the lung perfused by large collateral arteries. While pathophysiology differs significantly from Eisenmenger syndrome, there are important similarities in virtue of the significant right-to-left shunting and reduced pulmonary perfusion.

#### 9.1.2.1 Distinct differences between Eisenmenger syndrome and other types of PAH (Table 9.1)

Eisenmenger syndrome, especially in the presence of a post-tricuspid shunt, differs significantly from other types of PAH in terms

## Table 9.1 Differences between idiopathic pulmonary hypertension (iPAH) and Eisenmenger syndrome

|  | iPAH | Eisemenger syndrome |
|---|---|---|
| Associated genetic/ chromosomal disorders | No | Common (Down's syndrome) |
| Right ventriclular response |  |  |
|   Right ventricular dimensions | Dilation | Typically hypertrophy in post-tricuspid defects |
|   Right ventricular function | Rapid deterioration | Often preserved (VSD), quite stable |
| Cardiac output | Reduced | Substained by R-L shunting |
| Cyanosis |  |  |
|   Prevalence | When low-cardiac output and/or presence of PFO/ASD | The rule in Eisenmenger syndrome |
|   Severity | Rarely severe at rest | Often severe at rest even in stable patients |
| Haematologic effect | Rare unstudied haematologic manifestations | Secondary erythrocytosis |
| Systemic complications | Not common | Common (renal dysfunction) |
| Perception of limitation | Normal perception of limitation | Known to underestimate the degree of limitation as symptoms/limitations present from childhood |
| Medical therapy | Advanced therapies widely assessed in randomized trials. |  |
| Probable benefit in survival exists | Eisenmenger patients underrepresented in PAH clinical trials |  |
| Transplantation | Likely to benefit from transplantation | Slow progression, common systemic complications, complex cardiac disease. Not ideal candidates for transplantation |
| Prognosis | Poor, survival limited to few years after diagnosis | Not as poor, patients survive decades after diagnosis |

PAH: pulmonary arterial hypertension; R-L: right-to-left; PFO: patent foramen ovale; ASD: atrial septal defect of natural history and cardiac adaptation. While worse than in of the general population, the survival prospects in patients with Eisenmenger syndrome are much better than in idiopathic PAH (iPAH) or PAH related to connective tissue disease. This has important implications both in the clinical setting and when designing or interpreting clinical trials.

One reason for the substantial difference in mortality between Eisenmenger syndrome and other types of PAH is thought to be the response of the right ventricle to PAH. In iPAH and PAH related to connective disease, right ventricular dilation and dysfunction typically occurs, which progresses rapidly and relates to adverse outcome. In Eisenmenger patients with post-tricuspid shunts, the right ventricle typically does not dilate, but acquires a foetal-like phenotype by becoming hypertrophied with a preserved function, which may be more adapted to sustain an elevated afterload over a much longer period of time.

In Eisenmenger patients with pre-tricuspid defects (ASD), the response of the right ventricle to pressure overload tends to resembles that of iPAH: the right ventricle progressively dilates and systolic function becomes impaired. Even though long-term data are lacking, the natural history of these patients appears to resemble that of iPAH, with more rapid deterioration and worse survival prospects compared to Eisenmenger patients with a post-tricuspid shunt. The reason for the different response of the right ventricle may lie in the fact that PAH in these patients develops later in life, when the foetal right ventricular phenotype has been lost, or may be due to the absence of the large VSD which allows the left and right ventricle to work in unison reducing the load on the right ventricle. However, the 'disproportionate' response of the pulmonary circulation to an atrial communication and the pathophysiologic resemblance to iPAH raise legitimate concerns on whether these may be characterized as genuine 'Eisenmenger ASDs' or iPAH in the presence of a coexisting ASD.

Another important point of divergence between the Eisenmenger syndrome and other forms of PAH is the presence and extent of cyanosis. In iPAH and other forms of PAH, cyanosis is less common and less severe compared to Eisenmenger syndrome. It is usually the result of low cardiac output, and may be exacerbated by the presence of a patent foramen ovale or ASD. In patients with congenital heart disease, cyanosis occurs primarily as a result of significant right-to-left shunting through a large communication at rest and especially with exercise. Shunting in this setting contributes in maintaining cardiac output at rest and especially during mild-moderate exercise. This, however, occurs at the expense of significant hypoxia, increasing ventilation/perfusion mismatch and physiological dead space, which contribute to the marked ventilatory inefficiency and exercise intolerance, characteristic of Eisenmenger syndrome.

## 9.2 **Clinical manifestations of the Eisenmenger complex (Table 9.2)**

The clinical manifestations of Eisenmenger syndrome relate to the presence of PAH, cyanosis and the underlying cardiac disease. The raised pulmonary vascular resistance and significant right-to-left shunting result in severe exercise intolerance, which occurs early on in life and greatly impacts on quality of life. However, as this remains stable for many years, most Eisenmenger patients adapt their everyday 'normal' activities to their ability, thus minimising discomfort. Cyanosis, hypoperfusion and endothelial dysfunction also result in a high prevalence of systemic complications, such as kidney or liver dysfunction, which may independently affect prognosis.

---

**Table 9.2 Clinical manifestations and multiorgan involvement in Eisenmenger complex**

Exercise intolerance, dyspnoea, fatigue, dizziness

Hyperviscosity symptoms
• Headache, dizziness, visual disturbances, paresthesias (exclude iron deficiency and/or dehydration)

Severe cyanosis at rest and/or during exercise

Renal sysfunction

Haematologic involvement
• Secondary erythrocytosis
• Thrombocytopenia
• Iron deficiency

Thrombotic and bleeding diathesis
• Dilation of the pulmonary arteries, in situ thrombosis
• Haemoptysis, pulmonary haemorrhage
• Neoangiogenesis (GI, pulmonary, other bleeding)
• Cerebrovascular events

Arrhythmias
• Supraventricular tachycardias
• Ventricular tachycardia, sudden cardiac death

Rheumatologic complications
• Hyperuricemia and gout
• Hypertrophic osteoarthropathy, clubbing

Gastrointestinal complications
• Gallstones, cholecystitis

Bacterial infectious diseases
• Endocarditis
• Cerebral abscess
• Recurrent respiratory tract infection

Chronic cyanosis is also associated with significant haematologic changes. Secondary erythrocytosis is invariably present and is a physiological adaptation to chronic hypoxia aimed at increasing tissue oxygenation. Erythrocytosis in this setting is typically associated with a normal or low platelet count, and normal white cell count, making the term 'polycythaemia' inappropriate.

Bleeding diathesis is the result of thrombocytopenia, primary fibrinolysis and coagulation factor deficiencies. Haemoptysis is common in Eisenmenger syndrome and is the cause of death in 11–30% of patients, even though in most occasions, it is mild and self-limiting.

Increased red cell production and bleeding (e.g. haemoptysis, menses) commonly result in iron deficiency, which may cause or exacerbate hyperviscosity. Such caused symptoms are, in fact, uncommon in Eisenmenger syndrome and are usually caused or exacerbated by dehydration or iron-deficiency. Venesections (small amounts ≤ 500ml, with adequate volume replacement) are rarely indicated.

Eisenmenger patients are also prone to thrombotic events, in a paradoxical state of coexisting thrombotic and bleeding diathesis. Cerebrovascular events are common but may remain silent. Thrombosis of the central pulmonary arteries has been found in 20% of Eisenmenger patients and is thought to be in situ rather than embolic in origin. However, central pulmonary artery thrombi may become the source for peripheral pulmonary emboli, leading to pulmonary infarction and haemoptysis.

Myocardial dysfunction, valve disease and arrhythmias are also common in Eisenmenger syndrome and are the result of longstanding PAH, cyanosis and the underlying cardiac defect. Malignant arrhythmias are thought to be a major cause of death in this population, which is sudden in most cases.

### 9.2.1 **Prognosis**

Most Eisenmenger patients survive well into adulthood, decades after the diagnosis being established. In fact, while the 1-, 3-, and 5-year survival rates for iPAH are only 68%, 48% and 34% respectively, Eisenmenger patients live for decades after diagnosis and can reach the 4-5th decade of life. In a retrospective case-control study of 171 patients in our Institution, survival at 30, 40, 50, and 60 years of age was 98%, 94%, 74%, and 52%, respectively. Right ventricular function, complex congenital heart disease, functional class, and age of onset of clinical deterioration have been found to adversely affect the prognosis.

## 9.3 **Clinical management**

### 9.3.1 **Patient assessment and routine evaluation**

Eisenmenger patients are best followed in specialist centres with expertise both in ACHD and PAH (Table 9.3). Objective assessment

**Table 9.3 Evaluation of Eisenmenger patients and supportive treatment measures**

**Patient evaluation**

History-taking

- Exercise capacity
- Symptoms of hyperviscosity
- Bleeding or thrombotic events
- Syncopal or pre-syncopal episodes, arrhythmias
- Infection.

Physical examination

- Cyanosis, clubbing
- Nutritional status
- Evidence of heart or liver failure.

Investigations

- Chest radiogram
- ECG
- Blood tests (haemoglobin, ferritin, transferrin saturation, renal and hepatic function, electrolytes, thyroid function especially in Down syndrome patients, BNP)
- 6-minute walk test, cardiopulmonary exercise testing
- Transthoracic echocardiography
- High-resolution CT of the pulmonary arteries
- MRI.

**Supportive measures and precautions**

- Avoid dehydration
- Treat iron deficiency, avoid regular venesections
- Supplemental oxygen only when needed
- Avoidance of strenuous exercise and competitive sports
- Endocarditis prophylaxis
- Annual immunization against influenza and pneumococcal infections
- Careful planning of non-cardiac surgery
- Air travel appears safe, may use oxygen
- Avoidance of pregnancy: timely counselling and effective contraception.

of exercise tolerance should be performed periodically. The 6MWT is optimal for assessing severely impaired patients but inappropriate for mildly limited patients ('ceiling effect'), in which cardiopulmonary exercise testing may be more appropriate. Transthoracic echocardiography is used to assess cardiac anatomy, biventricular function, valvular competence and the presence of pericardial effusion. High-resolution chest computerized tomography and MRI provide additional information on the dimensions of the pulmonary arteries and the presence of in situ thrombosis, as well as cardiac and extracardiac lesions.

### 9.3.2 **Therapy**

The main goals of treatment are to improve quality of life, reduce complications, and increase survival.

#### 9.3.2.1 *Supportive measures and precautions*

Supportive care remains the mainstay of management of patients with Eisenmenger syndrome, and has the purpose of reducing symptoms and treating or preventing complications related to hypoxia, haematological or coagulation disorders, congestive cardiac failure, rhythm disturbances, and infection. Iron deficiency should be sought and treated wherever possible to avoid hyperviscosity symptoms and allow erythrocytosis appropriate to the degree of cyanosis. Routine venesections are to be avoided as they exacerbate iron deficiency and may increase the risk of stroke. Supplemental oxygen has a limited role in selected patients and only for nocturnal use, avoiding 'oxygen dependence'. Endocarditis prophylaxis is advisable for all cyanotic patients. Pregnancy remains at a prohibitively high risk (28% risk for death, mainly occurring in the post-partum period) and is generally contraindicated. General anaesthesia for non-cardiac surgery (intervention for gallstones, scoliosis, and, less commonly, cerebral abscess) carries a significant risk for these patients. It has been suggested that the bleeding risk may be reduced by preoperative phlebotomy if the hematocrit is more than 65%.

#### 9.3.2.2 *Heart failure medication, antiarrhythmics and implantable defibrillators*

Limited data are available on the benefit of heart failure medication, such as digitalis and diuretics, in Eisenmenger patients with signs of cardiac decompensation. Care should be taken when using diuretics to avoid dehydration, which may precipitate hyperviscosity and hypotension.

Arrhythmias of supraventricular or ventricular origin are frequent late sequelae of the Eisenmenger syndrome and may lead to clinical and haemodynamic deterioration or sudden cardiac death. Antiarrhythmics, especially amiodarone, are often used to control these arrhythmias, but evidence supporting this approach is lacking. The role of implantable defibrillators in this setting remains unknown but needs to be explored.

#### 9.3.2.3 *Anticoagulation*

The coexistence of haemoptysis and thrombosis makes clinical decision on anticoagulation arduous. No prospective studies have addressed the value of anticoagulants in this setting. Anticoagulation in Eisenmenger patients is supported by the finding of a high risk of thrombosis in the pulmonary arteries as well as by extrapolation of evidence supporting anticoagulation from studies in iPAH. Additional parameters such as the presence of intracavitary thrombi, arrhythmias, previous embolic phenomena versus the risk of haemorrhagic events, in particular haemoptysis, should be taken into consideration. Attention should be paid when assessing coagulation parameters in cyanotic patients with secondary erythrocytosis, as the amount of anticoagulant in vials used for blood collection should be reduced to match the decrease in plasma volume per unit of blood.

### 9.3.2.4 Disease-targeting PAH therapy

New 'advanced' therapies for PAH target vasoconstriction and proliferation of smooth muscle cells in the pulmonary arterial bed. This is achieved by acting on the three major pathways controlling these processes.

BREATHE-5 is the only large randomized, double-blind, placebo-controlled trial conducted in patients with Eisenmenger syndrome to date. In WHO class III patients, bosentan had a beneficial effect on exercise capacity and cardiopulmonary haemodynamics without compromising systemic oxygen saturation. The beneficial effects of bosentan on exercise capacity were maintained for up to 40 weeks in the open-label extension study. A small randomized trial of sildenafil in 10 Eisenmenger and 10 iPAH patients found a significant improvement in functional status, exercise capacity and pulmonary pressures in the Eisenmenger subgroup. Other large randomized trials using treprostinil, sildenafil, and sitaxentan have included a minority of patients with ACHD in their population. A minority of ACHD patients was also included in the recently published EARLY study assessing the effect of bosentan on PAH patients in functional class II, none of them had Eisenmerger syndrome.

A large number of non-randomized observational studies have reported a beneficial effect of advanced therapies in patients with ACHD, both in terms of haemodynamic and functional improvement, as well as quality of life. Data on longer follow-up are somewhat conflicting, however, some showing a persistent effect of advanced therapies at long-term, whereas others showing a loss of benefit after 1 year. Evidence of survival benefit of such therapies in Eisenmenger syndrome was recently published, based on a large non-randomized propensity score-based single institute cohort study. Little evidence on the use of combination therapy also exists and is only supported by observational studies.

### 9.3.2.5 Transplantation

Lung transplantation with repair of the underlying cardiac defect or heart and lung transplantation can be performed with an acceptable risk to eligible Eisenmenger patients. Transplantation is, however, restricted to highly symptomatic patients in whom life expectancy is considered short, and are thus likely to benefit from transplantation. As Eisenmenger patients tend to remain stable for many years, by the time transplantation is considered, they are poor candidates due to established multi-organ failure. This, together with the chronic shortage of donors, make the development of alternative therapies aimed at improving quality of life and survival of Eisenmenger patients, even more important.

### 9.3.2.6 Palliative Mustard procedure

A palliative Mustard procedure for patients with transposition of the great arteries, large VSD and PAH, consists of a surgical palliation employing an atrial switch procedure (Mustard or Senning), leaving the VSD open. This reduces cyanosis by redirection of flow, directing desaturated blood to the pulmonary artery and oxygenated blood to the aorta (streaming).

## 9.4 Conclusions

Eisenmenger syndrome is a perfect example of a disease previously considered untreatable and irreversible, now amenable to medical therapy, though not curative. While advanced PAH therapies have shown promising results in this population, supportive measures and precautions are as important in the management of these patients.

## 9.5 Acknowledgements

Dr Dimopoulos has been supported by the European Society of Cardiology. Dr Giannakoulas has been supported from the Hellenic Cardiological Society, the Hellenic Heart Foundation and the Cardiological Society of Northern Greece. The Royal Brompton Adult Congenital Heart Centre and Centre for Pulmonary Hypertension and Professor Gatzoulis have received support from the Clinical Research Committee, Royal Brompton Hospital, London and the British Heart Foundation.

## References

Ammash N, Warnes CA (1996) Cerebrovascular events in adult patients with cyanotic congenital heart disease. *J Am Coll Cardiol* **28**: 768–72.

Ammash NM, Connolly HM, Abel MD, Warnes CA (1999) Noncardiac surgery in Eisenmenger syndrome. *J Am Coll Cardiol* **33**: 222–7.

Bedard E, Dimopoulos K, Gatzoulis MA (2009) Has there been any progress made on pregnancy outcomes among women with pulmonary arterial hypertension? *Eur Heart J* **30**: 256–65.

Beghetti M, Galie N (2009) Eisenmenger syndrome a clinical perspective in a new therapeutic era of pulmonary arterial hypertension. *J Am Coll Cardiol* **53**: 733–40.

Broberg CS, Ujita M, Prasad S, et al. (2007) Pulmonary arterial thrombosis in eisenmenger syndrome is associated with biventricular dysfunction and decreased pulmonary flow velocity. *J Am Coll Cardiol* **50**: 634–42.

Daliento L, Somerville J, Presbitero P, Menti L, Brach-Prever S, Rizzoli G, Stone S (1998) Eisenmenger syndrome. Factors relating to deterioration and death. *Eur Heart J* **19**: 1845–55.

Diller GP, Dimopoulos K, Broberg CS, *et al.* (2006) Presentation, survival prospects, and predictors of death in Eisenmenger syndrome: a combined retrospective and case-control study. *Eur Heart J* **27**: 1737–42.

Diller GP, Dimopoulos K, Kafka H, Ho S, Gatzoulis MA (2007) Model of chronic adaptation: right ventricular function in Eisenmenger syndrome. *Eur Heart J* **9**: H54–60.

Diller GP, Gatzoulis MA (2007) Pulmonary vascular disease in adults with congenital heart disease. *Circulation* **115**: 1039–50.

Dimopoulos K, Diller GP, Koltsida E *et al.* (2008) Prevalence, predictors, and prognostic value of renal dysfunction in adults with congenital heart disease. *Circulation* **117**: 2320–8.

Dimopoulos K, Inuzuka R, Goletto S *et al.* (2010) Improved survival among patients with Eisenmenger Syndrome receiving advanced therapy for pulmonary arterial hypertension. *Circulation* **121**: 20–5.

Galie N, Beghetti M, Gatzoulis MA *et al.* (2006) Bosentan therapy in patients with Eisenmenger syndrome: a multicenter, double-blind, randomized, placebo-controlled study. *Circulation* **114**: 48–54.

Galie N, Rubin L, Hoeper M *et al.* (2008) Treatment of patients with mildly symptomatic pulmonary arterial hypertension with bosentan (EARLY study): a double-blind, randomised controlled trial. *Lancet* **371**: 2093–100.

Gatzoulis MA, Beghetti M, Galie N *et al.* (2007) Longer-term bosentan therapy improves functional capacity in Eisenmenger syndrome: Results of the BREATHE-5 open-label extension study. *Int J Cardiol*

Silversides CK, Granton JT, Konen E, Hart MA, Webb GD, Therrien J (2003) Pulmonary thrombosis in adults with Eisenmenger syndrome. *J Am Coll Cardiol* **42**: 1982–7.

Singh TP, Rohit M, Grover A, Malhotra S, Vijayvergiya R (2006) A randomized, placebo-controlled, double-blind, crossover study to evaluate the efficacy of oral sildenafil therapy in severe pulmonary artery hypertension. *Am Heart J* **151**: 851 e1–5.

Spence MS, Balaratnam MS, Gatzoulis MA (2007) Clinical update: cyanotic adult congenital heart disease. *Lancet* **370**: 1530–2.

Territo MC, Rosove MH (1991) Cyanotic congenital heart disease: hematologic management. *J Am Coll Cardiol* **18**: 320–2.

Wood P (1958) The Eisenmenger syndrome or pulmonary hypertension with reversed central shunt. *Br Med J* **2**: 755–62.

## Chapter 10

# Respiratory causes of pulmonary hypertension

Tamera Jo Corte and S John Wort

### Key points

- Pulmonary hypertension (PH) associated with lung disease or hypoxaemia is a distinct subgroup of PH
- PH related to respiratory disease is often mild-to-moderate in severity. However, PH may be out-of-proportion and moderate to severe to the underlying lung disease in a minority of patients. The presence of PH is associated with poorer survival
- Multiple mechanisms often contribute to the pathophysiology of PH related to lung disease including: chronic hypoxaemia, destruction of the pulmonary vasculature, true vascular remodelling, in situ thrombosis, and upset of the pulmonary angiogenesis/angiostasis balance
- Management is based upon treatment of the under-lying disorder(s), their complications, and reversal of resting hypoxaemia. There have been no successful randomized-controlled trials for specific PH therapies in respiratory patients, so no routine specific PH therapy is recommended. However, uncontrolled trials and case-series for endothelin-receptor antagonists and vasodilators have been encouraging. Larger placebo-controlled trials are underway.

## 10.1 Introduction and classification

PH is defined haemodynamically by right heart catheter (RHC) measurements of a mean pulmonary arterial pressure (mPAP) $\geq 25$ mmHg at rest, with a pulmonary capillary wedge pressure $\leq 15$mmHg and pulmonary vascular resistance $\geq 3$ Wood units.

The classification of PAH was revised at the World Symposium on Pulmonary Arterial Hypertension in Dana Point (PAH, Table 10.1) where PAH was divided into five main groups. PAH associated with lung disease or hypoxaemia was identified as a distinct subgroup, with subcategories including PAH related to chronic obstructive pulmonary disease (COPD), interstitial lung disease (ILD), and a third sub-group including sleep-disordered breathing, alveolar hypoventilation disorders, chronic exposure to high altitude, and developmental abnormalities. Multi-systemic disorders such as sarcoidosis, LAM and LCH are included in the last 'miscellaneous' group.

In general PAH related to respiratory disease is mild-to-moderate, and survival depends on the severity of the underlying lung disease, rather than the PAH *per se*. However, where PAH develops these patients have a worse prognosis. In some conditions such as COPD, ILD and sarcoidosis, there appears to be an outlying minority group with PAH 'out of proportion' to their lung disease. These groups may represent patients with a more 'vascular' phenotype.

## 10.2 **Diagnosis of PAH in respiratory disease**

Recognition of PAH may be delayed, as it is often masked by the clinical picture of the underlying respiratory disease. Symptoms including dyspnoea and fatigue are common to both PAH and advanced respiratory disease. Physical signs reflective of PAH (such as a loud pulmonary component of the second heart sound) are often difficult to hear in respiratory disease. Signs of right heart failure (including peripheral oedema) are generally late findings.

### 10.2.1 **Right heart catheter**
RHC remains the gold standard for the diagnosis of PAH. It allows the direct measurement of the pulmonary artery pressure (PAP), as well as the right atrial, ventricular pressure, and the pulmonary arterial wedge pressure. RHC is a moderately invasive procedure, requiring hospital admission, and so a number of non-invasive investigations are often used in the assessment for PAH.

### 10.2.2 **Echocardiography**
Continuous Doppler flow echocardiography allows estimation of the systolic PAP from the maximal velocity of the tricuspid regurgitation jet. It is not possible to estimate the systolic PAP in the absence of tricuspid regurgitation. Although echocardiography is the most reliable non-invasive method to diagnose PAH, its accuracy is lower in patients with chronic lung disease. However, echocardiography

**Table 10.1 Dana point classification of pulmonary arterial hypertension**

1. Pulmonary arterial hypertension (PAH)
   1.1 Idiopathic PAH
   1.2 Heritable
       1.2.1 BMPR2
       1.2.2 ALK1, endoglin (with or without hereditary hemorrhagic telangectasia)
       1.2.3 Unknown
   1.3 Drug and toxin induced
   1.4 Associated with:
       1.4.1 Collagen tissue diseases
       1.4.2 HIV infection
       1.4.3 Portal hypertension
       1.4.4 Congenital heart diseases
       1.4.5 Schistosomiasis
       1.4.6 Chronic haemolytic anemia
   1.5 Persistent pulmonary hypertension of the newborn
   1.6 Pulmonary veno-occulsive disease (PVOD) and/or pulmonary capillary haemangiomatosis (PCH)

2. Pulmonary hypertension with left heart disease
   2.1 Left-sided atrial or ventricular heart disease
   2.2 Left-sided valvular heart disease

3. Pulmonary hypertension associated with lung diseases and/or hypoxemia
   3.1 Chronic obstructive pulmonary disease
   3.2 Interstitial lung disease
   3.3 Other pulmonary diseases with mixed restrictive and obstructive pattern
   3.4 Sleep disordered breathing
   3.5 Alveolar hypoventilation disorders
   3.6 Chronic exposure to high altitude
   3.7 Developmental abnormalities

4. Chronic thromboembolic pulmonary hypertension (CTEPH)

5. Pulmonary hypertension with unclear multifactorial mechanisms
   5.1 Hematologic disorders: myeloproliferative disorders, splenectomy
   5.2 Systemic disorders: sarcoidosis, pulmonary Langerhans cell histiocytosis, lymphangioleiomyomatosis, neurofibromatosis, vasculitis
   5.3 Metabolic disorders: glycogen storage disease, Gaucher disease, thyroid disorders
   5.4 Others: tumoral obstruction, fibrosing mediastinitis, chronic renal failure on dialysis.

does complement RHC in the assessment of PH, as it provides other, structural cardiac information.

### 10.2.3 **Natriuretic peptides**

Brain natriuretic peptide (BNP) is released in response to atrial and ventricular wall stretch. Plasma BNP concentrations are elevated in pulmonary arterial hypertension, and PH associated with lung disease (including COPD and ILD). There is some evidence to suggest that elevated BNP is also a marker of poor prognosis in patients with chronic lung diseases.

### 10.2.4 **Pulmonary function**

Patients with chronic lung disease with PH have lower $PaO_2$ and gas transfer levels than those without PH. However, there is poor correlation between spirometric volumes and PAP, as PH can develop at any stage of the underlying disease.

### 10.2.5 **Exercise testing**

Cardiopulmonary exercise tests (CPET) may be useful to identify early, or exercise-induced PH, as a cause of exercise-limitation in these patients with underlying lung disease. However, often patients are unable to perform a CPET, and six-minute walk testing (6MWT) is used instead. 6MWT is a reproducible test. Patients with lung disease and PH have lower 6MWT distance, and lower end-exercise $SpO_2$, and these findings portend poorer prognoses.

### 10.2.6 **Imaging**

The main and segmental pulmonary artery size may be measured on computerized tomography (CT) scanning (Figure 10.1). There is little data to support the use of CT scanning in the diagnosis of PH in patients with lung disease.

Cardiac MRI provides the most accurate measurement of right ventricular mass and ejection fraction. Its role in the diagnosis of PH in this patient group is promising, but needs further study.

## 10.3 **Management of PAH associated with respiratory disease**

Management of PH related to respiratory disease includes treatment of the underlying disorder(s). Hypoxaemia correlates to some extent with PH, and supplemental oxygen is recommended to reverse resting hypoxaemia in these patients. Full assessment and treatment of co-morbidities (including diastolic heart failure, pulmonary emboli and obstructive sleep apnoea) is important.

Specific PH therapy is not routinely recommended for these patients, as there have been no successful placebo-controlled trials

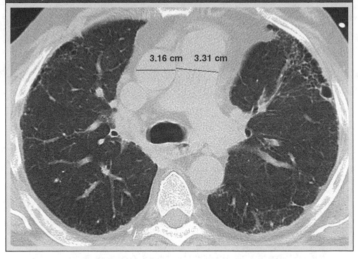

Fig 10.1 **CT** scan of a patient with idiopathic pulmonary fibrosis and pulmonary hypertension (with dilatation of the main pulmonary artery, compared to the aorta)

3.16 cm    3.31 cm

of disease-targeted PH therapies in this patient group. There is a potential risk of increasing pulmonary shunting and ventilation-perfusion mismatch particularly with pulmonary vasodilators. However, uncontrolled trials and case-series have shown promising results with endothelin-receptor antagonists (ERA) and sildenafil, and placebo-controlled trials are currently underway.

137

## 10.4 Pathophysiology of pulmonary hypertension associated with respiratory disease

The pathophysiology of PH related to lung disease is complex, with multiple mechanisms contributing to its pathogenesis (Figure 10.2).

### 10.4.1 Chronic hypoxia

Hypoxic pulmonary vasoconstriction (HPV) largely occurs in the 'muscular' pre-capillary arterioles. Hypoxia results in the development of free radicals, inflammatory cell recruitment and cytokines, which in turn lead to HPV. This adaptive response allows redirection of blood flow to better-ventilated lung, minimizing ventilation-perfusion mismatch. Although chronic hypoxia is an important contributing factor to increased vascular resistance in chronic lung disease, PH occurs in patients without hypoxaemia, suggesting that PH in lung disease is not attributable to hypoxia alone.

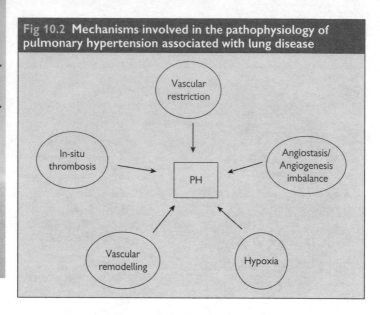

Fig 10.2 Mechanisms involved in the pathophysiology of pulmonary hypertension associated with lung disease

### 10.4.2 **Pulmonary vascular destruction**

The destruction of the pulmonary vascular bed that occurs in chronic lung diseases such as COPD and ILD results in raised pulmonary vascular resistance. Traditionally this was thought to be the primary factor in the development of PH. However, the poor correlation between the extent of the lung disease (on CT or pulmonary function tests) and PH suggests that it is only partly responsible.

### 10.4.3 **Pulmonary vascular remodelling**

Pulmonary vascular remodelling results from increase in cell number in all components of the vessel wall. This leads to a narrowed lumen and increase in vascular resistance proportional to radius. Although the formation of plexiform lesions, characteristic of severe pulmonary arterial hypertension, are not generally seen in respiratory diseases (Table 10.2, Figure 10.3), true remodelling of resistance vessels has been reported. Furthermore, pathogenetic mediators known to be important in vascular remodelling in PAH, such as endothelin-1 (ET-1), are implicated in some respiratory diseases.

### 10.4.4 **In-situ thrombosis**

*In situ* thrombosis refers to thrombosis occurring within the pulmonary arteries and arterioles, often at sites of endothelial damage. This process contributes to the narrowing of the pulmonary vessels and complex vascular remodelling. It is frequently seen in pulmonary arterial hypertension, but is also thought to occur in PH associated with lung disease. An imbalance in circulating and tissue coagulation factors contributes to *in situ* thrombosis in these patients.

**Table 10.2** Features of pulmonary vascular remodelling in patients with pulmonary arterial hypertension and pulmonary hypertension related to respiratory disease

| | Idiopathic pulmonary arterial hypertension | Pulmonary hypertension associated with lung disease |
|---|---|---|
| Adventitial changes | Prominent | Present |
| Medial smooth muscle hypertrophy | Prominent | Prominent |
| Distal smooth muscle neomuscularization | Prominent | Prominent |
| Intimal proliferation | Common | Mild |
| Monoclonal endothelial cell proliferation | Present | Not described |
| In situ thrombosis | Common | Present |
| Plexogenic lesions | Common | Not described |

## 10.5 Specific respiratory disorders—prevalence and pathogenesis and treatment

### 10.5.1 Chronic obstructive pulmonary disease

It is estimated that mPAP rises by 0.28–0.6 mmHg/year in COPD, so a significant proportion will develop PH over their lifetime. PH is usually mild-to-modest in severity, except for a group of outliers with more significant PH out-of-proportion to their underlying airflow limitation. PH does confer a worse prognosis, being an independent factor for both mortality and frequency of COPD exacerbations.

#### 10.5.1.1 Pathogenesis

Traditionally, PH was thought to be due to pulmonary vascular destruction, and chronic hypoxia. However, PH is not related to the extent of emphysema, occurs independently of hypoxia and is not ameliorated by oxygen replacement. Other mechanisms, must, therefore, be considered particularly for disproportionate PH. Potential mechanisms include: transient hypoxia (on exercise, at night, and during exacerbations); hypercapnia, which leads to vasoconstriction; and cigarette smoke, which may cause direct endothelial dysfunction. Finally, ET-1 may contribute to the development of PH in COPD. Plasma ET-1 levels are elevated in acute exacerbations and with nocturnal desaturation.

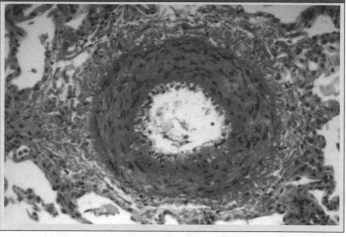

**Fig 10.3** Histopathology of pulmonary artery in pulmonary hypertension (expansion of all three layers of the pulmonary artery is present in PH)

Furthermore, levels of ET-1 have been shown to correlate with echocardiographic systolic PAP.

### 10.5.1.2 Management

Currently, there is no recommended therapy for PH in COPD patients, excepting supplemental oxygen. Controlled trials are warranted to determine optimal treatment.

Long-term supplemental oxygen stabilizes and sometimes reverses the progression of PH, although PAP may not return to normal. Supplemental oxygen is recommended at >16 hrs/day for patients with daytime resting hypoxia. In patients without daytime hypoxia, there is insufficient evidence to recommend the use of nocturnal oxygen for the prevention or treatment of PH in COPD patients.

There has been one randomized study of the ERA, bosentan, on cardiopulmonary hemodynamics in patients with severe COPD (but not PH). Bosentan treatment did not improve 6MWT distance, and was associated with poorer oxygenation and quality of life. There was however a reduction in pulmonary vascular resistance.

### 10.5.2 Interstitial lung disease

PH is not uncommon in ILD, especially in severe disease. In idiopathic pulmonary fibrosis (IPF) patients referred for lung transplantation, reported prevalence is 32–46%. PH develops over time in these patients, as demonstrated by the rise in prevalence of PH in IPF patients from 33% at initial assessment to up to 85% immediately prior to transplantation. However, PH is not confined to patients with advanced lung disease. There is a poor correlation between the severity of PH and the extent of the underlying lung disease. PH is associated with poorer prognoses in IPF. Systolic PAP >50 mmHg on echocardiography is associated with a median survival of 0.7 yrs, compared to 4.8 yrs for a sPAP of ≤35 mmHg.

### 10.5.2.1 Pathogenesis

A broad pathogenetic distinction can be made between secondary and disproportionate PH. Fibrotic vascular ablation and chronic hypoxic vasoconstriction appear to account for PH secondary to advanced fibrosis but are less applicable to disproportionate PH. In patients with disproportionate PH, potential factors include molecular mediators common to PH and ILD and intermittent hypoxia (especially during sleep and exercise).

Historically, PH secondary to ILD was attributed to fibrotic ablation of pulmonary vessels, and the subsequent elevation in pulmonary vascular resistance. Vascular ablation is likely to play a major part in the development of PH in end-stage fibrosis but is less relevant to the sub-group of patients with disproportionate PH.

Chronic hypoxia is important in the development of secondary PH in patients with slowly progressive chronic conditions but does not explain the presence of PH in ILD patients with limited fibrosis or normoxia. Even in advanced ILD, resting hypoxia is a late finding and is, thus, unlikely to play a primary causative role for PH. Longer-standing intermittent nocturnal or exercise-induced hypoxia may play a crucial role in the development of disproportionate PH.

Several cell mediators are involved in the pathogenesis of both lung fibrosis and PH (e.g. 5-lipoxygenase, transforming growth factor-$\beta$, TNF-$\alpha$ and ET-1), suggesting an overlap in the pathogenesis of these disorders.

### 10.5.2.2 Management

Historically, treatment has focused on reversal of hypoxia and treatment of the underlying respiratory condition. Although no specific data available in ILD, supplemental oxygen is recommended in light of the likely pathogenetic role of hypoxia. The benefit of reversing intermittent hypoxia (at night, or on exercise) is unknown.

Vasodilators have been used cautiously in ILD patients, due to the potential risk of worsened gas exchange. Shunt fraction and hypoxemia increases with IV prostaglandin-I2 but not nitric oxide or sildenafil, which cause selective pulmonary vasodilation. Limited IPF data suggests a clinical and hemodynamic benefit of sildenafil. A single dose of sildenafil acutely improves pulmonary hemodynamics and gas exchange. Three small case-series demonstrated a small improvement in echocardiographic parameters and exercise capacity in IPF patients treated with sildenafil for three months.

The role of ERAs in PH associated with ILD is not widely studied. The 'Bosentan use in Interstitial Lung Disease' (BUILD)-1 study demonstrated no benefit of bosentan over placebo in IPF. There was a non-significant trend towards improvement for patients taking bosentan that may reflect the presence of a responsive subgroup (perhaps those with underlying vascular decompensation). In a small open-label IPF study bosentan was well-tolerated, but not associated with changes in clinical or physiological parameters at three months. Further studies are warranted to determine the effect of specific PH therapy in ILD.

### 10.5.3 **Sarcoidosis**

Sarcoidosis, a multi-system granulomatous disorder, commonly affects the lungs, and may result in progressive pulmonary fibrosis. PH is a well-recognized complication of sarcoidosis, occurring in <5% of patients. PH is more common in patients with advanced disease, and has been reported in up to 75% of sarcoidosis patients awaiting lung transplantation. PH is associated with a poor prognosis in sarcoidosis patients.

The severity of the PH does not correlate well with the severity of the underlying lung disease. In fact, PH may be more severe when it occurs in the absence of fibrotic pulmonary sarcoidosis. This suggests that there are other factors apart from the underlying lung disease contributing to the pathogenesis of PH.

#### *10.5.3.1 Pathogenesis*

In contrast to other ILD, extrinsic compression of the large pulmonary arteries by sarcoid lymphadenopathy may result in increased pulmonary vascular resistance. Other potential causes of PH in sarcoidosis include fibrotic destruction of the pulmonary vascular bed, hypoxic pulmonary vasoconstriction, pulmonary veno-occlusive disease, porto-pulmonary-PH, cardiac sarcoidosis, and a primary pulmonary granulomatous vasculopathy.

The role of hypoxaemia is not clearly defined in PH in sarcoidosis. In advanced sarcoidosis, patients with PH have higher oxygen requirements. However, one study showed no relationship between pulmonary pressures and the level of hypoxaemia suggesting that factors other than hypoxia play a role in the development of PH in sarcoidosis. ET-1 levels are increased in the urine, plasma and bronchoalveolar lavage fluid in some sarcoid patients, and may contribute to the development of PH.

#### *10.5.3.2 Management*

There is little data to guide the management of PH in sarcoidosis. There are conflicting reports regarding corticosteroids, with some describing improvement, and others worsening of PH. One study describes an improvement following corticosteroid treatment in patients without pulmonary fibrosis, but no effect in patients with pulmonary fibrosis. Case reports of successful PH therapy include vasodilators such as epoprostenol, nitric oxide, calcium channel blockers and ET-1 receptor antagonists such as bosentan. Placebo-controlled studies are underway to determine the effect of PH specific therapies in sarcoidosis.

### 10.5.4 Cystic fibrosis (CF)

CF, a common genetic disorder occurring in 1 of every 2,000 live births, results in progressive cystic lung disease, eventually leading to respiratory failure, PH, cor pulmonale and death. PH occurs in up to 40% of those with severe, stable lung disease, and is less common in patients with better pulmonary function. In CF patients awaiting transplantation, PH is a poor prognostic determinant (median time to death or transplantation 15 months compared to 33 months in those without PH). Cor pulmonale is often viewed as a pre-terminal event.

#### 10.5.4.1 Pathogenesis

PH is considered to be due to the underlying destruction of the lung parenchyma, and to hypoxaemia related pulmonary vasoconstriction. Pulmonary pressures are inversely related to pulmonary function ($FEV_1$), and are associated with lower oxygen saturation levels (at rest, following exercise, and at night) independent of pulmonary function. This suggests that resting and intermittent hypoxaemia do play a role in the pathogenesis of PH in CF patients.

PH is more commonly observed in patients with chronic infection with B. multivorans, an organism associated with poor prognosis. This association raises the possibility that chronic inflammation, or inflammatory mediators (eg interleukin-6, interleukin-1 and tumour necrosis factor-$\alpha$) may play a role in the pathogenesis.

#### 10.5.4.2 Management

Early assessment for PH is recommended, particularly in patients with cor pulmonale, deteriorating pulmonary function, B. multivorans infection and chronic hypoxaemia. No studies have specifically addressed the role of therapy for PH in CF. Aggressive therapy of the underlying lung disease, and prompt referral for pulmonary transplantation are crucial in CF patients with PH, as survival is reduced in these patients. Appropriate oxygen supplementation is recommended, although further work is required to determine whether oxygen replacement (especially on exercise and at night) modifies or prevents the development of PH in CF patients.

### 10.5.5 Neuromuscular and chest wall disorders

Neuromuscular disorders (such as muscular dystrophy) and other disorders impairing chest wall expansion (including kyphoscoliosis and obesity) may lead to PH and eventually cor pulmonale. The prevalence of PH is unknown, and relates to the severity of the underlying disorder.

### 10.5.5.1 Pathogenesis

The reduction in ventilatory capacity in these disorders, leads to hypoxaemia, hypercapnia and acidosis and subsequent pulmonary vasoconstriction and eventual PH. Nocturnal hypoventilation (particularly in REM sleep) often precedes daytime respiratory failure in these patients, and is associated with nocturnal oxygen desaturation and daytime hypercapnia. The severity of the PH correlates with the severity of the sleep-disordered breathing in these patients.

### 10.5.5.2 Management

Treatment of PH focuses upon correction of the underlying disease process. Correction of hypoxaemia does improve pulmonary haemodynamics, however may worsen hypercapnia, and is therefore not recommended alone. Nocturnal ventilation, either by non-invasive ventilation or tracheostomy and intermittent positive pressure ventilation, improves hypoxaemia, and there is limited data suggesting that it may partly reverse PH in these patients.

## 10.5.6 **Sleep-disordered breathing**

Sleep-disordered breathing includes obstructive sleep apnoea (OSA), and obesity hypoventilation syndrome (OHS). OSA is extremely common, occurring in 9% of men, and 4% of women, characterized by nocturnal hypopneas and apneas and subsequent excessive daytime somnolence, snoring, and observed apnoeic events. OHS, usually occurs in patients with OSA, and is characterized by resting hypoxia and daytime hypercapnia with compensated respiratory acidosis. OSA alone may cause mild PH, but rarely leads to PH in the absence of daytime hypoxaemia. OSA may be a cofactor for PH in patients with other underlying respiratory disorders (especially COPD).

### 10.5.6.1 Management

Therapy of PH in this setting is focused on treatment of the underlying disorder, including weight loss and continuous positive airway pressure nocturnal ventilation (with or without supplemental oxygen). No studies have directly assessed the affect of such therapy on PH, but patients with PH have the greatest symptomatic benefit from therapy.

## 10.5.7 **Pulmonary histiocytosis X**

Pulmonary histiocytosis X (HCX), an ILD often associated with cigarette smoking, has a variable prognosis. Many improve following smoking cessation, but a minority progress to pulmonary fibrosis. PH is almost universal in patients with HCX awaiting lung transplantation. Pulmonary arterial pressures are higher in patients with HCX than in other chronic lung diseases of similar severity. Pressures are similar to those seen in idiopathic pulmonary arterial hypertension, and are not associated with pulmonary function or hypoxaemia. The exercise limitation seen in HCX is linked to pulmonary vascular dysfunction rather than ventilatory limitation.

### 10.5.7.1 Pathogenesis

PH in HCX is related to intrinsic involvement of the pulmonary vasculature, rather than secondary to the parenchymal lung disease. Diffuse pulmonary vasculopathy is present at histopathology, with medial hypertrophy, intimal and subintimal fibrosis and proliferation, and luminal narrowing of both the pulmonary arteries and veins. These changes may be directly associated with Langerhans' cell granulomata, but are often geographically distinct, possibly related to the production of cytokines and growth factors released from the granulomata.

### 10.5.7.2 Management

There is little data on the treatment of PH in this HCX. While the similarities to idiopathic pulmonary arterial hypertension suggest a role for specific therapy in this disorder, there are no trials to support such practice. Additionally, the prominent venous involvement in HCX suggests that pulmonary vasodilators (such as prostacyclin therapy) may be unsafe, as in patients with veno-occlusive disease. Pulmonary transplantation remains an important consideration in such cases.

## 10.5.8 **Lymphangioleiomyomatosis (LAM)**

LAM, a disorder primarily affecting women, is characterized by the proliferation of abnormal smooth-muscle-like cells leading to thin walled pulmonary cysts, central lymphatic abnormalities, and abdominal tumours (angiomyolipomas).

PH is a recognized complication of LAM, and is primarily seen in patients referred for pulmonary transplantation. Resting PH is uncommon (<10%) in LAM patients with moderate functional impairment. However, over 50% of LAM patients develop PH on moderate exercise, and the rise in pulmonary pressure is associated with hypoxaemia. This suggests that hypoxaemia-mediated pulmonary vasoconstriction may contribute to the pathogenesis of PH in LAM.

### 10.5.8.1 Management

No data is available for the specific treatment of PH in LAM. Early referral for pulmonary transplantation is paramount. Appropriate oxygen supplementation (at rest and exercise) is also recommended to prevent hypoxaemia, and possibly prevent or modify the development of PH.

## 10.6 **Summary**

PH is associated with poorer outcomes in patients with underlying lung disease. Although PH in this context has often been considered mild-to-moderate, it may occur out of proportion to the underlying lung disease. Pathophysiologic mechanisms are complex, and cannot be entirely attributable to destruction of the lung parenchyma and resultant hypoxaemia. Management of PH in these patients is focused upon treatment of the underlying lung disease, and reversal of hypoxaemia. There is no supporting evidence for the routine use of specific PH therapies in these patients at present. However, there is an urgent need for controlled trials of therapies used to treat pulmonary arterial hypertension to establish safety and efficacy for patients with respiratory diseases.

# References

Baughman RP, Engel PJ, Meyer CA, Barrett AB, Lower EE (2006) Pulmonary hypertension in sarcoidosis. *Sarcoidosis Vasc Diffuse Lung Dis* **23**: 108–16.

Behr J, Ryu JH (2008) Pulmonary hypertension in interstitial lung disease. *Eur Respir J* **31**: 1357–67.

Chaouat A, Naeije R, Weitzenblum E (2008) Pulmonary hypertension in COPD. *Eur Respir J* **32**: 1371–85.

Fartoukh M, Humbert M, Capron F *et al.* (2000) Severe pulmonary hypertension in histiocytosis X. *Am J Respir Crit Care Med* **161**: 216–23.

Fauroux B, Hart N, Belfar S *et al.* (2004) Burkholderia cepacia is associated with pulmonary hypertension and increased mortality among cystic fibrosis patients. *J Clin Microbiol* **42**: 5537–41.

Fraser KL, Tullis DE, Sasson Z, Hyland RH, Thornley KS, Hanly PJ (1999) Pulmonary hypertension and cardiac function in adult cystic fibrosis: role of hypoxemia. *Chest* **115**: 1321–8.

Han MK, McLaughlin VV, Criner GJ, Martinez FJ (2007) Pulmonary diseases and the heart. *Circulation* **116**: 2992–3005.

Lee TM, Chen CC, Shen HN, Chang NC (2008) Effects of pravastatin on functional capacity in patients with chronic obstructive pulmonary disease and pulmonary hypertension. *Clin Sci (Lond)*.

Nathan SD (2008) Pulmonary hypertension in interstitial lung disease. *Int J Clin Pract Suppl* 21–8.

Nunes H, Humbert M, Capron F *et al.* (2006) Pulmonary hypertension associated with sarcoidosis: mechanisms, haemodynamics and prognosis. *Thorax* 61: 68–74.

Polomis D, Runo JR, Meyer KC (2008) Pulmonary hypertension in interstitial lung disease. *Curr Opin Pulm Med* **14**: 462–9.

Presberg KW, Dincer HE (2003) Pathophysiology of pulmonary hypertension due to lung disease. *Curr Opin Pulm Med* **9**: 131–8.

Simonneau G (2004) Proceedings of the 3rd World Symposium on Pulmonary Arterial Hypertension. Venice, Italy, June 23–25, 2003. *J Am Coll Cardiol* **43**: 1S–90S.

Simonneau G, Robbins IM, Beghetti M *et al.* (2009) Updated clinical classification of pulmonary hypertension. *J Am Coll Cardiol* **54**: S43–54.

Taveira-DaSilva AM, Hathaway OM, Sachdev V, Shizukuda Y, Birdsall CW, Moss J (2007) Pulmonary artery pressure in lymphangioleiomyomatosis: an echocardiographic study. *Chest* **132**: 1573–8.

## Chapter 11

# Other causes of pulmonary hypertension

Sara Goletto, Ryo Inuzuka and Koichiro Niwa

> **Key points**
>
> - Patients with HIV and pulmonary arterial hypertension (PAH) have an increased risk of death compared to those without. Bosentan has been shown to improve functional capacity without interfering with antiretroviral drug plasma concentrations
> - Chronic schistosomiasis is one of the most common causes of PAH in endemic areas. A high index of suspicion is necessary when patients from such areas are presented with symptoms suggesting possible pulmonary hypertension
> - In patients with portal hypertension, the risk of developing pulmonary arterial hypertension increases with the duration of the disease. Screening for PAH is recommended if liver transplantation is considered
> - The prevalence of PAH amongst patients with sickle cell disease is about 30% and significantly reduces survival. Right heart catheterization is recommended In suspected cases to confirm the diagnosis of PAH and rule out pulmonary venous hypertension due to left heart disease, which is often present in this population.

Other than the previously described causes of pulmonary hypertension (PH) in the preceding chapters, further causes need consideration. These include HIV infection, schistosomiasis, portal hypertension and sickle cell disease (Table 11.1). The prevalence of some of these diseases is high in some parts of the world. It is important to diagnose PH when present in these conditions, as it impacts significantly on clinical course. However, signs and symptoms of PH often overlap with those of the primary disease, presenting a diagnostic challenge. Advanced therapies in this setting have been shown to have some beneficial effects albeit assessed only in small studies.

**Table 11.1** Other causes of pulmonary hypertension

| Causes of PH | Prevalence of PH |
|---|---|
| PAH associated with | |
|   Portal hypertension | 2–6% |
|   HIV infection | 0.5% |
|   Drugs and toxins (especially anorectic agents) | 3% in anorectic agents use |
|   Other causes | |
|     Thyroid disorders | 35–50% |
|     Glycogen storage disease (type 1) | Only few cases |
|     Gaucher disease | 7% |
|     Hereditary hommorrhagic telangiectasia | 15% |
|     Hemoglobinopathies (Sickle cell anemia) | 30% |
|     Myeloproliferative disorders | 15% |
|     Splenectomy | 50% in hemolytic disease |
| PAH associated with PVOD or PCH | 100% (definition) |
| Miscellaneous | |
|   Sarcoidosis | 5% |
|   Langerhance cell histiocytosis X | Unknown but 100% in and stage |
|   Lymphangiomatosis | Unknown |
|   Schistosomiasis | 7.5–21.6% |

PAH = pulmonary arterial hypertension, PCH = pulmonary capillary hemangiomatosis, PH = pulmonary hypertension, PVOD = pulmonary veno-occlusive disease.

## 11.1 **HIV infection**

- *Prevalence*: There are an estimated 40 million patients with HIV disease worldwide, 0.5% of them have pulmonary arterial hypertension (PAH). In fact, HIV-related PAH seems to account for approximately 10% of all PAH causes (Sitbon, 2008). Prevalence and severity of PAH are not related to the stage of HIV infection, but its occurrence may relate to the duration of HIV infection

- *Mechanism*: Histologically, plexogenic arteriopathy is found in the majority of cases. The underlying mechanism of PAH in HIV is unclear, but is unlikely to be due to direct infection of the pulmonary endothelium. HIV antigens have been shown to trigger abnormal apoptosis and proliferation of endothelial cells

- *Clinical impact*: The presenting symptoms of PAH in HIV patients are shortness of breath resulting from right ventricular dysfunction. Patients with HIV and PAH have a two-fold increased risk of death compared with those without (Opravil et al., 1997). However, routine screening for PAH is not recommended due to the low prevalence of PAH in HIV patients (McLaughlin *et al.*, 2009)

- *Treatment*: The potential interaction of antiretroviral therapy (ART) with HIV-PAH remains controversial. Although ART induces endothelial dysfunction in in-vitro studies and potentially exacerbates PAH, a retrospective study demonstrated improved hemodynamics and survival with ART. Intravenous epoprostenol improves functional class, exercise capacity and hemodynamic parameters. However, the risk of catheter-related sepsis remains an issue in patients with immunosuppression. Some case reports have demonstrated the effectiveness of oral sildenafil. However, drug interaction between sildenafil and antiretroviral drugs occurs and dosing must be adjusted accordingly. Bosentan has been shown to benefit HIV-PAH patients in terms of functional class and 6 minute walk test, without interfering with antiretroviral drug plasma concentrations. Anticoagulation in HIV-PAH has to be done carefully due to the risk of thrombocytopenia and associated liver dysfunction (Sitbon, 2008).

## 11.2 Schistosomiasis

- *Prevalence*: Schistosomiasis is the third-leading parasitic disease in the world affecting more than 300 million people. It is the most common cause of PH in the endemic areas (ex; sub-Saharan Africa, eastern South America, the Caribbean Islands, east Asia, and parts of China) (Butrous *et al.*, 2008). It is caused by trematode flatworms called *Schistosoma*, whose life cycle involves several developmental stages. The infection can be contracted whilst walking and swimming in infested freshwater. The organisms penetrate the skin and travel via the bloodstream to their target organs where they deposit their eggs: *S. haematobium* in the urinary tract, *S. mansoni* and *S. japonicum*, in the intestinal and hepatic circulatory system. PH relates to chronic schistosomiasis rather than acute infection. The exact prevalence of PH caused by schistosomiasis is unknown, although small studies have reported rates of 7.5% to 21.6%, and when present, it carries a grave prognosis

- *Pathology*: PH could occur as a consequence of several mechanisms. Elevated proinflammatory cytokines due to chronic immunological response might directly cause endothelial dysfunction, vasoconstriction and smooth muscle proliferation (Butrous *et al.*, 2008). Portal hypertension secondary to liver fibrosis resulting from delayed hypersensivity reaction to the deposited eggs, can also lead to PH. Furthermore, the development of portal-systemic collateral circulation due to portal hypertension allows the eggs to shunt from the liver to the lungs, and thus induces a local immunological response

- *Diagnosis*: Symptoms and chest radiographs do not have distinctive features. The diagnosis depends on detection of eggs in urine or fecal samples using microscopy (that can disappear after previous treatment). Serological tests can be used as a marker of previous exposure. Signs of portal hypertension with periportal fibrosis seen on abdominal imaging and maintained liver function is characteristic in schistosomiasis

- *Treatment*: Although anti-infective agents like praziquantel are effective treatment for acute infections, their efficacy on chronic schistosomiasis is unknown. The use of advanced therapies for PH in this setting has not been established.

## 11.3 **Portal hypertension**

- *Definition*: Portopulmonary hypertension refers to PAH in association with portal hypertension (portal pressure > 10 mmHg). Liver cirrhosis is the most common cause of portopulmonary hypertension. Mild increase in pulmonary artery pressure due to increased cardiac output is often observed in patients with cirrhosis. However, portopulmonary hypertension is distinct from this cirrhotic hyperdynamic status and the usual diagnostic criteria for PAH apply, namely: mean pulmonary arterial pressure > 25 mmHg at rest, pulmonary vascular resistance > 240 dyness cm-5 and left ventricular end-diastolic pressure < 15mmHg

- *Prevalence*: The prevalence of portopulmonary hypertension is 2 to 6% among patients with portal hypertension. Conversely, portal hypertension accounts for approximately 9% of PAH. The risk of developing PAH increases with the duration of portal hypertension. However, the underlying mechanism by which portal hypertension results in pulmonary hypertension is not fully established (Wells *et al.*, 2008)

- *Clinical impact*: The most common symptom is that of progressive dyspnoea on exertion. Signs of right heart failure due to PAH, such as jugular venous distention, oedema and ascites, are less specific as they are also seen in decompensated cirrhosis. PAH significantly increases the risks of any surgery and in particular, of liver transplantation. Screening for PH is recommended if liver transplantation is considered

- *Treatment*: Several open-label studies have shown that intravenous epoprostenol improves hemodynamics and exercise capacity in patients with portopulmonary hypertension. Recently, bosentan, despite its potential hepatotoxicity, has been shown to be safe and effective in patients with portopulmonary hypertension. Sildenafil has also been reported to decrease pulmonary vascular resistance. Liver transplantation maybe a treatment option for selected patients. Mild to moderate PAH is often reversible after liver transplantation, whereas severe PAH is not, and thus associated with high mortality. The use of anticoagulants in this setting is controversial because of an increased risk of variceal bleeding (Hoeper *et al.*, 2004).

## 11.4 Sickle cell disease

- *Prevalence*: Sickle cell disease is one of the most common autosomal recessive disorders worldwide with about 30 million individuals being affected. This is the major cause of PAH associated with hemolytic anemia. The reported prevalence of PH amongst adult patients with sickle cell disease is approximately 30%

- *Mechanism*: Severe chronic hemolysis can induce vasoconstriction, endothelial dysfunction, platelet activation and smooth muscle proliferation through reduction of the available nitric oxide and elevation in endothelin-1 levels. Other important causative factors include a pro-coagulant state, asplenia, chronic lung disease, nocturnal hypoxemia, iron overload, and left heart disease (diastolic failure), many of which frequently co-exist in these patients

- *Clinical impact*: The symptoms of PH resemble those of anemia, making the diagnosis difficult and often delayed. Patients with anemia usually become symptomatic with relatively low values of mean pulmonary artery pressure (30–40 mm Hg). The presence of PH, even in mild forms, significantly reduces the survival (reported 2-year mortality rates of 40–50%). Screening for PH with transthoracic Doppler echocardiography, performed at rest, at least 2 weeks after an acute painful crisis and 4 weeks after an acute chest syndrome or blood transfusion, is recommended every year to enable early detection and timely therapy (Lee *et al.*, 2007) (McLaughlin *et al.*, 2009). Right heart catheterization is recommended in suspected cases to confirm the diagnosis of PH and rule out pulmonary venous hypertension due to left heart disease often present in this population (Machado, 2007)

- *Treatment*: Hydroxycarbamide and red-cell transfusions are indicated to reduce hemolysis and prevent PH. Treatment of causal factors is also important, such as iron chelation for iron overload, heart failure treatment for left ventricular dysfunction, oxygen for hypoxemia, anticoagulation for thromboembolism and C-PAP for sleep apnea. Advanced therapies including sildenafil and oral L-arginine (the substrate for nitric oxide synthesis) have been shown to improve 6-minute walk distance, the pulmonary systolic pressure and the plasma NT pro-BNP levels in small studies.

## 11.5 **Conclusion**

We have discussed rare causes of PAH affecting patients in the developed and developing world and having clear adverse impact on clinical outcome. Greater awareness of PAH as a complication of these conditions and its timely diagnosis may facilitate available therapies, and thus improve prospects for these patients.

# References

Butrous G, Ghofrani HA, Grimminger F (2008) Pulmonary vascular disease in the developing world. *Circulation* **118**: 1758–66.

Hoeper MM, Krowka MJ, Strassburg CP (2004) Portopulmonary hypertension and hepatopulmonary syndrome. *Lancet* **363**: 1461–8.

Lee MT, Rosenzweig EB, Cairo MS (2007) Pulmonary hypertension in sickle cell disease. *Clin Adv Hematol Oncol* **5**: 645–53, 585.

Machado RF (2007) Sickle cell anemia-associated pulmonary arterial hypertension. J Bras Pneumol **33**: 583–91.

McLaughlin VV, Archer SL, Badesch DB et al. (2009) ACCF/AHA 2009 expert consensus document on pulmonary hypertension: a report of the American College of Cardiology Foundation Task Force on Expert Consensus Documents and the American Heart Association. *Circulation* **119**: 2250–94.

Opravil M, Pechere M, Speich R et al. (1997) HIV-associated primary pulmonary hypertension. A case control study. Swiss HIV Cohort Study. *Am J Respir Crit Care Med* **155**: 990–5.

Sitbon O (2008) HIV-related pulmonary arterial hypertension: clinical presentation and management. *Aids* **22**: Suppl 3, S55–62.

Wells JT, Runo JR, Lucey MR (2008) Portopulmonary hypertension. *Hepatology* **48**: 13–5.

## Chapter 12

# Pregnancy and pulmonary arterial hypertension

Elisabeth Bédard

---

**Key points**

- Pregnancy in women with pulmonary arterial hypertension (PAH) is associated with prohibitive maternal mortality
- Early advice on pregnancy risks, including contraception is paramount
- Women with PAH who become pregnant warrant a multidisciplinary approach and should be followed in a tertiary centre with expertise on PAH
- Targeted PAH therapies should be considered before decompensation occurs.

---

## 12.1 Introduction

Pregnancy in women with pulmonary arterial hypertension (PAH), including idiopathic (iPAH), in association with congenital heart disease (CHD-PAH) or PAH due to other causes (oPAH), is known to be associated with a high maternal mortality. The physiological changes that occur during pregnancy and the peripartum seem to be poorly tolerated in these patients and their offspring, who is also at high risk of significant complications. Therefore, counselling of affected women of childbearing age about the potential risks of pregnancy is mandatory. Women with PAH who become pregnant and choose to continue their pregnancy warrant a multidisciplinary approach. During the past decade or so, the management of high-risk pregnancies has improved and new advanced therapies for the treatment of PAH have been developed, improving overall quality of life and prognosis for these patients (Drenthen *et al.*, 2007, Bedard *et al.*, 2009). This chapter reviews major issues regarding pregnancy in woman with PAH.

## 12.2 **Hemodynamic changes during pregnancy**

Table 12.1 summarizes the major hemodynamic perturbations occurring during pregnancy. Most women with PAH have abnormal right ventricular size and function prepartum. Pregnancy-induced haemodynamic changes add to the burden of an impaired right ventricle, and can trigger further deterioration in right ventricular systolic function, sometimes irreversible. Systemic vasodilatation and the increase in cardiac output may enhance right-to-left shunting and exacerbate pre-existing hypoxia in patients with CHD-PAH, leading to further pulmonary vasoconstriction.

Significant volume overload can occur during labour and immediately after delivery caused by uterine contractions, leading to transfusion of a large amount of blood into the circulation, and by decompression of the inferior vena cava. Further haemodynamic stress can occur at that stage, when hypercarbia and acidosis may increase pulmonary hypertension acutely, leading to refractory right heart failure Weiss et al., 1998, Siu et al., 2001, Bonnin et al., 2005,

| Table 12.1 Physiological changes during pregnancy | | |
|---|---|---|
| **Parameter** | **Changes** | **Comments** |
| Plasma volume | ↑ up to 50% | • 2nd to stimulation of the angiotensin renin aldosterone system induced by estrogens<br>• ↑ in plasma is greater than ↑ in red blood cells, creating "physiological anaemia" |
| Peripheral vascular resistance | ↓ 20–30% | 2nd to:<br>• Hormonal activity<br>• ↑ Pg, BNP, NO<br>• ↑ temperature produced by the foetus<br>• Low resistance circulation in utero |
| Systolic BP | ↓ 5–10 mmHg | ↓ starting during 1st trimester, peak at mid pregnancy, back to normal before week 40th |
| Diastolic BP | ↓ 10–15 mmHg | |
| Heart rate | ↑ 10–15 bpm | Maximum during 3rd trimester |
| Cardiac output | ↑ up to 50% | • ↑ as soon as 5th week, max 24th week<br>• 1st trimester: 2nd to ↑ stroke volume; 3rd trimester: 2nd to ↑ in heart rate<br>• 3rd trimester: ↓ up to 30% in supine position |

Uebing *et al.*, 2006). Episodes of hypotension, either secondary to blood loss and hypovolemia or due to vasovagal reaction, are potentially fatal in this population. Although most haemodynamic changes induced by pregnancy will have return to prepregnancy levels within 2 weeks, they persist for several months after delivery (Clapp *et al.*, 1977) occasionally leading to persistent right heart failure and even late death.

## 12.3 Counselling

To avoid an unplanned and dangerous pregnancy, women should be counselled in early adolescence about the risk of pregnancy, both to themselves and to their baby. Advice about contraception is essential. Ideally, both a cardiologist with expertise in PAH and an interested obstetrician/gynaecologist should be involved. Information should include:

- Contraception
- Life expectancy
- Risks for the mother
- Risks for the foetus
- Level of surveillance, need for treatment and anticipated hospitalization required should pregnancy occur.

### 12.3.1 Contraception

Because of the prohibitive risks mentioned below, pregnancy should be strongly discouraged in patients with PAH. Early contraception advice should be provided in all women of child-bearing age and termination should be considered if pregnancy occurs. Highly effective methods with low rate of side effects (such as venous thromboembolism) should be selected; the following methods are therefore recommended:

- Depot injection of progestogen and subcutaneous implants with slow release of progesterone (e.g. Nexplanon®)
- Hormonal intrauterine system (Mirena® coil).

Vasoagal reaction may occur during insertion of a coil; the latter should be inserted in operating room with anaesthesiologist available. Other methods such as condoms and combined oral contraceptive should be avoided in this population because of their significant failure rate. Moreover, risk of thromboembolic event is increased with the combined pill which contains oestrogen.

### 12.3.2 Life expectancy

Women with PAH who wish to start a family should be aware that they might not be there to look after their child. Although there has been improvement in survival with targeted therapies for PAH (Galie *et al.*, 2009), life expectancy in patients with iPAH remains limited to few years after diagnosis. Patients with Eisenmenger syndrome have better prognosis than iPAH or oPAH, but nearly one third of them will have died by the age of 40 years (Cantor et al., 1999).

### 12.3.3 Risks for the mother

Parturients with PAH are at high risk of severe cardiovascular complications, such as:

- Right heart failure
- Pulmonary hypertension crisis
- Thomboembolic events
- Bleeding
- Arrhythmias
- Death.

Mortality rates among parturients with PAH remain prohibitively high, albeit they might have decreased in the last decade compared to previous era (Bedard et al., 2009) (Figure 12.1).

Indeed, published reports of pregnant patients with PAH from 1978 to 1996 revealed a maternal mortality of 30% in iPAH, 36% in Eisenmenger syndrome, and 56% in oPAH (Weiss et al., 1998), while reports from 1997 to 2007 showed a mortality of 17%, 28% and 33%, respectively (Bedard et al., 2009). Better management and the use of targeted therapies for PAH may explain these improved results.

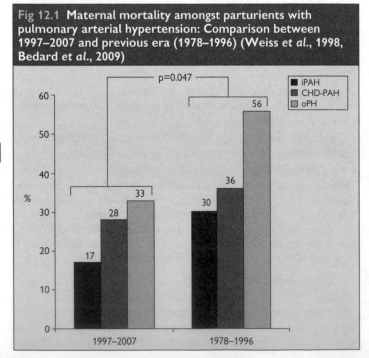

Fig 12.1 **Maternal mortality amongst parturients with pulmonary arterial hypertension: Comparison between 1997–2007 and previous era (1978–1996) (Weiss et al., 1998, Bedard et al., 2009)**

The majority of deaths amongst parturients with PAH occur in the peripartum period, mainly within the first month following delivery. This underscores the ongoing challenge of parturients with PAH to cope with the haemodynamic changes related to pregnancy, further exaggerated by acute changes during delivery and the postpartum. CHD-PAH patients, mostly with Eisenmenger syndrome, are also predisposed to systemic complications such as bleeding and thrombotic diathesis, arrhythmias, and multiorgan involvement, which may contribute to the increased maternal mortality observed.

### 12.3.4 **Risks for the foetus**

Foetuses and newborns of mothers with PAH also have significant risk of complications, including (Drenthen *et al.*, 2007):

- Small-for-gestational-age birth weight/intrauterine growth retardation
- Premature birth
- Respiratory distress syndrome
- Intraventricular hemorrhage (when mother is on anticoagulation therapy).

Neonatal outcomes are even worse when the mother has poor functional class (>2), cyanosis or receives anticoagulants (Siu *et al.*, 2002). Parturients with PAH therefore require increased intensity of antepartum foetal surveillance, including more frequent foetal echocardiograms.

## 12.4 **Management of pregnant women with PAH**

If a patient opts out of continuing with her pregnancy, she should be looked after in a tertiary center with experienced cardiologists, obstetricians, anaesthetists, and neonatologists. More frequent visits during pregnancy are advised, and hospitalization at the beginning of the third trimester might facilitate the management and preparation of the multidisciplinary team. A detailed plan including timing and mode of delivery should be discussed in advance.

### 12.4.1 **Mode of delivery**

The optimal mode of delivery (vaginal versus caesarean section) in patients with PAH remains controversial. However, vaginal delivery is associated with smaller shifts in blood volume, fewer clotting or bleeding complications, and a lower risk of infection (Uebing *et al.*, 2006, Steer *et al.*, 2008). Caesarean section may become necessary in cases of maternal haemodynamic deterioration or foetal distress requiring urgent delivery. Some centres advocate elective caesarean section, which allow for optimal preparation and avoidance of emergency situation after a prolonged unsuccessful labour. In any case, a close surveillance and a low threshold for intervention with early signs of maternal or foetal distress are recommended.

### 12.4.2 **Anaesthesia**

Regional anaesthesia, either by epidural with small incremental doses or by combined-epidural anaesthesia, could be the safest method in patients with PAH. General anaesthesia is known to depress cardiac contractility (volatile agents), increase pulmonary vascular resistance (positive pressure ventilation) and may result in an increase in pulmonary arterial pressure during laryngoscopy and intubation (Price et al., 2007). Therefore, general anaesthetics in patients with PAH may increase risk of complications (Bedard et al., 2009, Bonnin et al., 2005). Anaesthesia/analgesia should be offered early during labour to avoid increase in cardiac output associated with contraction and pain. Moreover, it should be performed by an experienced anaesthetist.

### 12.4.3 **Peripartum monitoring**

Cardiac rhythm, blood pressure and arterial oxygen saturation should be monitored carefully throughout the peripartum (Kiely et al., 2006); an arterial line and a central venous catheter for monitoring of right atrial pressure should be considered in patients with PAH. Insertion of a pulmonary artery catheter to monitor pulmonary arterial pressure remains controversial. Complications such as pulmonary artery rupture have been reported, and there is no evidence that it improves outcomes in these patients (Barash et al., 1981). Therefore, invasive pulmonary arterial pressure monitoring should not be used routinely in parturients with PAH and should be considered only in selected cases.

### 12.4.4 **Thromboprophylaxis**

Pregnancy increases x 6 the risk of thromboembolic events in all normal parturients. This risk is even higher in pregnant women with PAH; low-dose subcutaneous heparin prophylaxis is generally recommended in this population. However, the level of anticoagulation should be discussed within the multidisciplinary team for each case separately; specially in Eisenmenger syndrome, which is associated with both thrombotic and bleeding complications. Moreover, some patients may require higher levels of anticoagulation (e.g. patients with history of thromboembolic events or atrial fibrillation). Pulmonary thrombrosis causing peripartum death has been reported; timely consideration of thromboprophylaxis is mandatory and should be discussed with the patient.

## 12.5 **Peripartum targeted therapies for PAH**

The effects of targeted PAH therapies (such as nitric oxide, calcium channel blockers, prostacyclin analogues, endothelin-receptor antagonists and phosphodiesterase inhibitors) on parturients with PAH remain unknown. In most case reports published in the past ten years, targeted PAH therapies were administered late, as a last resort when parturients were already haemodynamically unstable (Bedard et al., 2009). Instead, targeted therapies should be considered earlier during pregnancy and labour, before haemodynamic deterioration occurs.

- **Inhaled nitric oxide (NO)** has been shown to cause an acute drop in pulmonary vascular resistance in Eisenmenger syndrome (Budts et al., 2001), iPAH (Leuchte et al., 2004), and chronic pulmonary thromboembolic disease (Ulrich et al., 2006). Its administration during labour and delivery may potentially reduce the risk of developing severe RV failure or pulmonary hypertensive crisis

- **Calcium channel blockers** are safe during pregnancy (Magee et al., 1996) and may prevent preterm labour (Simhan et al., 2007), a common complication in patients with PAH. However, calcium channel blockers may be beneficial only in acutely vasoreactive patients with iPAH, which represent less than 10% of iPAH patients (Sitbon et al., 2005)

- **Prostacyclin analogues** (nebulized iloprost or intravenous) have been used successfully in some pregnant women with PAH (Elliott et al., 2005). Nebulized iloprost offers the advantage of avoiding the risk of line infections. Prostacyclin analogues should be considered as valuable therapeutic options in this setting

- **Endothelin-receptor antagonist** bosentan may have teratogenic effects (Madsen et al., 2001) and is, thus, contraindicated during pregnancy

- **Phosphodiesterase inhibitor** sildenafil has not been associated with any deleterious effects on the mother or offspring in animal studies and in two case reports on humans (Villanueva-Garcia et al., 2007). Sildenafil can be administered orally; it represents an attractive option in this population.

159

## 12.6 **Conclusion**

Maternal mortality in parturients with PAH remains prohibitively high. Early advice on pregnancy risks and appropriate contraception is, thus, paramount. When a patient with PAH becomes pregnant, follow-up in a tertiary centre by a multidisciplinary team with experience in high-risk pregnancies appears mandatory. Hospitalization during the third trimester should be considered and a detailed plan for the management should be discussed in advance and agreed with the patient. Targeted PAH therapies and effective thromboprophylaxis must be considered before patients decompensate or thrombotic complications ensue.

# References

Barash PG, Nardi D, Hammond G et al. (1981) Catheter-induced pulmonary artery perforation. Mechanisms, management and modifications. *J Thorac Cardiovasc Surg* **82**, 5–12.

Bedard E, Dimopoulos K, Gatzoulis MA (2009) Has there been any progress made on pregnancy outcomes among women with pulmonary arterial hypertension. *Eur Heart J* **30**, 256–65.

Bonnon M, Mercier FJ, Sitbon O et al. (2005) Severe pulmonary hypertension during pregnancy: mode of delivery and anaesthetic management of 15 consecutive cases. *Anesthesiology* **102**, 1133–7; discussion 5A–6A.

Budts W, Van Pelt N, Gillyns H, Gewillig M, Van de Werf F, Janssens S (2001) Residual pulmonary vasoreactivity to inhaled nitric oxide in patients with severe obstructive pulmonary hypertension and Eisenmenger syndrome. *Heart* **86**, 553–8.

Cantor WJ, Harrison DA, Moussadki JS et al. (1999) Determinants of survival and length of survival in adults with Eisenmenger syndrome. *Am J Cardiol* **84**, 677–81.

Clapp JF III, Capeless E (1997) Cardiovascular function before, during, and after the first and subsequent pregnancies. *Am J Cardiol*, **80**, 1469–73.

Drenthen W, Pieper PG, Roos–Hesselink J et al. (2007) Outcome of pregnancy in women with congenital heart disease: a literature review. *J Am Coll Cardiol,* **49**, 2303–11.

Elliott CA, Stewart P, Webster VJ et al. (2005) The use of iloprost in early pregnancy in patients with pulmonary arterial hypertension. *Eur Respir J* **26**, 168–73.

Galie N, Manes A, Negro L, Palazzini M, Bacchi-Reggiani ML, Branzi A (2009) A meta-analysis of randomized controlled trials in pulmonary arterial hypertension. *Eur Heart J* **30**, 394–403.

Kiely D, Elliot C, Webster V, Stewart P (2006) Pregnancy and pulmonary hypertension: new approaches to the management of life-threatening condition. In: Steer P, Gatzoulis MA, Baker P (Eds) *Heart Disease and Pregnancy*. London, RCOG Press.

Leuchte HH, Schwaiblmair M, Baumgartner RA, Neurohr CD, Kolbe T, Behr J (2004) Hemodynamic response to sildenafil, nitric oxide, and iloprost in primary pulmonary hypertension. *Chest* **125**, 580–6.

Madsen KM, Neerhof MG, Wessale JL, Thaete LG (2001) Influence of ET(B) receptor antagonism on pregnancy outcome in rats. *J Soc Gynecol Investig* **8**, 239–44.

Magee LA, Schick B, Donnenfield AE et al. (1996) The safety of calcium channel blockers in human pregnancy: a prospective, multicentre cohort study. *Am J Obstet Gynecol* **174**, 823–8.

Price LC, Forrest P, Sodhi V et al. (2007) Use of vasopressin after Caesarean section in idiopathic pulmonary arterial hypertension. *Br J Anaesth* **99**, 552–5.

Simhan HN, Caritis SN (2007) Prevention of preterm delivery. *N Engl J Med* **357**, 477–87.

Sitbon O, Humbert M, Jais X *et al.* (2005) Long-term response to calcium channel blockers in idiopathic pulmonary arterial hypertension. *Circulation* **111**, 3105–11.

Siu SC, Colman JM, Sorensen S *et al.* (2002) Adverse neonatal and cardiac outcomes are more common in pregnant women with cardiac disease. *Circulation* **105**, 2179–84.

Steer PJ (2005) Pregnancy and contraception. In: Gatzoulis MA, Swan L, Therrien J, Pantely GA (Eds) *Adult congenital heart disease: a practical guide.* Oxford, BMJ Publishing/Blackwell Publishing.

Uebing A, Steer PJ, Yentis SM, Gatzoulis MA (2006) Pregnancy and congenital heart disease. *BMJ* **332**, 401–6.

Ulrich S, Fischler M, Speich R, Popov V, Maggiorini M (2006) Chronic thromboembolic and pulmonary arterial hypertension share acute vasoreactivity properties. *Chest* **130**, 841–6.

Villanueva-Garcia D, Mota-Rojas D, Hernandez-Gonzalez R *et al.* (2007) A systematic review of experimental and clinical studies of sildenafil citrate for intrauterine growth restriction and pre-term labour. *J Obstet Gynaecol* **27**, 255–9.

Weiss BM, Zemp L, Seifert B, Hess OM (1998) Outcome of pulmonary vascular disease in pregnancy: a systematic overview from 1978 through 1996. *J Am Coll Cardiol* **31**, 1650–7.

# Index

Page numbers in *italic* indicate figures and tables.

163